Jon & Karen

now had time only for each other.
The more time they spent together,
the more intimate they became
in every area of their lives.
It wasn't long until their sexual
attraction for each other became the
focus of their hours together.
She and Jon had already found
that the nebulous term "going too
far" had no absolute line.
The more passionate their kissing,
the more inadequate it seemed as an
expression of their love.
Even so, she and Jon were confident
that they could stop "before it
was too late." After all, they had
asked God to protect and help
them, hadn't they?

Karen's Choice

JANICE HERMANSEN

LIVING BOOKS
Tyndale House Publishers, Inc.
Wheaton, Illinois

First printing, January 1985
Library of Congress Catalog Card Number 84-52344
ISBN 0-8423-2027-X, paper
Copyright 1985 by Janice Hermansen
Printed in the United States of America

CHAPTER

1

KAREN entered Flanders Hall and wrinkled her nose. The building reeked of musty wallpaper and furniture polish. "This place gives me the creeps!" she muttered. It seemed almost haunted with old memories and faded glory. She frowned at the threadbare rugs and overstuffed furniture. For a moment, she could almost imagine her parents courting in the lobby.

Wryly amused, she recalled their glowing remarks and naive assumptions about their alma mater. "This old school just ain't what she used to be," she sang under her breath. Times changed, people changed, but dear old Flanders Hall had remained almost exactly as her mother remembered it when she had lived there twenty-five years ago.

Back then, "Bible" was the main subject taught at Wellington Christian College; curfew was seven o'clock in the evening; and physical contact between couples, as innocent as holding hands, carried a threat of suspension. The list of rules went on and on back then, but her parents hadn't seemed to mind.

"Ah, nostalgia!" Karen rolled her eyes, and charged full-steam up the four flights of stairs to her room. "Fifty, fifty-one, fifty-two ...," she counted under her breath as he tried to imagine what her mother was like as a young woman. *Beautiful, of course—and in love,* she thought romantically. She stopped to rest on the third-floor landing.

I just wish I were as sure about love as Mom and Dad were, she told herself, a worried frown flitting across her face. *Charles.* There he was again, crowding into her thoughts. *Do I really love him?* Her mind seesawed briefly, and then, shrugging away her doubts, she bolted up the remaining steps.

A few moments later, as she unlocked her door, she wondered why she'd bothered to hurry. The mere thought of entering her room depressed her. Karen despised the mustard-yellow walls with the matching carpet, drapes, and bedspreads. She found it hard to believe that someone had actually color-coordinated a room in that horrible shade. She and Tricia, her roommate, had tried to decorate, but the posters and stuffed animals only looked out of place.

With a discouraged sigh, Karen sat at her desk and prepared to study. She closed her eyes for a moment to escape the ugly surroundings and visualized her bedroom back home. Dainty, flowered wallpaper, a white, textured ceiling with tiny gold-star sparkles, the glossy dark wood floor with fluffy blue throw rugs, white shuttered windows. . . .

Within a few moments, she was wallowing miserably in homesickness. *And then there's Charles* . . . she reminded herself despondently as she opened her eyes and gazed at his picture. His longish dark hair complemented his gentle brown eyes, which crinkled when he smiled.

They'd grown up together in Myrtle Point, a small town on the Oregon coast. After dating regularly all through high school, they'd gone steady during her senior year, even though Charles was many miles away at Wellington College, in Seattle, Washington. And now that they were both attending Wellington after that miserable year apart, Charles had asked her to marry him.

And like a dope, I said yes, Karen thought darkly as she examined her engagement ring. It *was* beautiful, she had to admit. All sparkly and reflecting the light in a thousand ways, it evoked delighted, if envious comments from the other girls in the dorm.

She felt a sudden urge to throw the ring out the window. *What's wrong with me?* she asked herself as she had countless times before. She reminded herself that her friends admired Charles even more than they did the ring.

Karen supposed they were right. Charles did have some good points. He was a Christian, and he was reliable, hard-working, sincere, eager to please her. . . . Her list faltered. *What else?* Karen asked herself. She thought hard, trying to remember more of his good qualities. She scowled in frustration as she realized that for some reason, he didn't have enough. Not for her, anyway. *But why? What do I want?* she argued silently with her disquieting thoughts. *Maybe I'm just confused by being away from home—or maybe I expect too much.*

She sighed and glanced up at her calendar, suddenly missing her parents and hometown almost more than she could bear. *How many days 'til Christmas?* she wondered and began counting the squares remaining in November.

As she flipped the page to December, she pictured her mom and dad, the huge fir tree that would scrape the living room ceiling, old friends, caroling and hot chocolate, the little kids who'd stumble through the Christmas program at church. . . .

The door opened with a loud squeak, shattering her daydream. Karen frowned inadvertently as her roommate entered.

"What's the matter? Did I do something wrong?" Tricia asked as she carefully placed a large brown box on her bed.

"No, I guess I'm just homesick—again." Karen eyed the parcel with interest. It had to be a care package from Tricia's mother.

"Why don't you check your mailbox? Look what I got!" Trish attacked the strapping tape. "Where are the scissors? Quick! I smell food!" The two girls nearly tore the package apart in their haste to sample its contents.

"Maybe I *will* take a walk to the post office," Karen said, as she helped herself to a handful of oatmeal raisin cookies. "Not that I'm expecting anything," she added offhandedly, her wistfulness barely concealed.

"Where's your faith?" Tricia teased.

"No faith involved—just facts." Karen grabbed her coat and headed for the door.

"I'll bet there's a letter for you," Trish called after her.

That's Trish, the eternal optimist, Karen thought, repressing a smile. She admired her roommate for her steady disposition and quick sense of humor. Tricia never seemed to let circumstances get her down.

Karen reflected on the many differences between them. People often remarked that the two roommates were a study in contrasts. Trish could have been a model. Her shoulder-length golden hair always did what it was supposed to, and she could wear any style of clothing with her tall, leggy figure. Her beautiful fresh face with its sparkling blue eyes and light freckles belonged on a magazine cover.

Karen surveyed herself in the hall mirror. *No model material here,* she decided, though she knew she was pretty. She wore a petite size five, and stretched her bones to reach the five foot mark. Her waist-length curly brown hair defied her attempts to style it—especially on important occasions. She had soft, smoky brown eyes, which tended to reflect her serious personality. She quickly brushed her hair and then skipped lightly down the stairs.

Once outside, she stared up at the scrawny, bare-limbed trees outlined against the sullen sky.

She felt a sudden, freezing bite in the air, and pulling her coat tightly around her, she quickened her pace. The wind began to tug at her coat, and tiny slivers of rain teased her to hurry. *Maybe there will be a letter. Do I dare hope?* she wondered. Letters from home never seemed to come as often as Karen needed them. Splatter-drops pelted her as she sprinted the remaining distance to the student union building.

Once inside, Karen leaned against a wall as she caught her breath. *This place is a madhouse today!* she thought as she noted the scores of college kids crammed wall-to-wall. Everyone seemed to have chosen the same place as shelter from the impending rainstorm.

She watched students playing Ping-Pong and air hockey. Others feverishly worked the video games, while the stereo blared. A few people nonchalantly dance-stepped, though dancing was still technically against the rules at Wellington. Couples lounged on sofas and stared into each other's eyes, oblivious to the crowd around them. *They should sit up straighter,* Karen thought in disgust.

Closing her eyes for a moment, she listened to the chink of coins being dropped into the vending machines and then the satisfying clunk of the delivered goods, the padding of tennis shoes paired with the staccato beat of fashionable boots, the slamming of metal against metal—oh, the mailboxes! Karen's eyes opened in astonishment for she'd completely forgotten why she'd come.

She hurried over to the post office and peered

into her tiny mailbox window. There it was! She could scarcely believe her good fortune as she excitedly fumbled with the combination, and at last managed to open the tricky lock. As she held the bulky letter she glanced around, hoping for a secluded place to enjoy her treasure.

Finding nothing better, Karen sat down on a nearby staircase and read hurriedly, skimming the news. Her father, the pastor of a small coun-try church, wrote about a humorous incident in a wedding he had performed. "You should have been there," he said. "It was an absolute riot!"

Karen chuckled. She would have loved to have witnessed the scene. She turned to her mom's portion of the letter. "Uh, oh," she thought as she read on.

"I've noticed that you haven't mentioned Charles much in your letters or phone calls," her mother pointed out. "Are you still engaged? He's a wonderful person, Karen. You know we love him dearly. But are you sure about marriage, honey? You're young, and you have plenty of time to decide on such an important step. And really, we'd like to see you finish college first. I don't mean to be nosey—I just love you. . . ." The words on the page blurred and Karen closed her eyes to hold back the threatened flood.

She wasn't fooling anyone—not even her mother. And least of all, Karen knew she wasn't fooling herself. *I don't love Charles,* she admit-ted. *Not enough to marry him.* She stared hard at the glittering engagement ring and finally yanked it off, but strangely that made her feel worse. She sighed. *Maybe I really do love him—I don't know. And if I tell Charles how I feel, I'll hurt him terribly,* she told herself miserably as she replaced the ring on her finger.

She resolutely pushed the subject out of her mind, and turned back to her letter. Her mother had also included newspaper clippings as well as some snapshots of friends. She'd even sent pictures of their home and church, the high school, the county fairgrounds, and the beach. "You forgot the grocery store, Mom," Karen giggled, "and how about the post office?" She turned to the news clippings and perused them carefully.

A sudden shadow darkened the page she was reading. Startled, she glanced up and faintly recognized the tall, blond-haired young man, though she couldn't quite place him. She thought maybe he was a junior.

"Hi, I'm Jon," he introduced himself. "I have some classes with you—American history and French." He smiled uncertainly as if he were waiting for an answer.

"Hi," she finally managed to say, "I'm Karen, I–I think I remember seeing you before...." *What does he want?* she wondered uncomfortably.

"Is that a letter from home?" he asked, pointing at her thick envelope. Without waiting for an invitation, he sat down beside her.

Well! Karen thought, somewhat overwhelmed by his approach. *He's got a lot of nerve!* But he almost seemed as though he wanted to share her "care package," so she responded, "Yes, and they sent pictures, too. Would you like to see them?"

"Sure!" he leaned forward and eagerly took the

snapshots. "What's this—your old high school? And who are these people?"

"Some friends . . . and that's my mom and dad—" The figures blurred as she tried to wipe away sudden tears. "I'm sorry," she apologized. She was furious and embarrassed at her inability to control her emotions, especially in front of someone she hardly knew. "I get so homesick that it's just ridiculous!"

Jon reached over and patted her shoulder comfortingly. "Hey, don't feel bad about crying," he said. "In fact, I think it's kind of neat."

"Why?" Karen eyed him in disbelief. "What's so great about being homesick?" Her question was punctuated with a few sniffles.

Jon paused for a moment as though he were carefully choosing his words. Finally he answered, "If you didn't care about your parents, there wouldn't be anything to cry about. And if they didn't care about you, there wouldn't be any need to send pictures and letters. I really envy you." He hunched his shoulders and gazed reflectively at his tennis shoes.

Karen was shocked by Jon's candid comments. Charles would never be that open, not even with her. She swallowed hard and asked, "Don't you have a family?"

"Sure," he said, "I have a family—or pieces of one, anyway. My folks divorced a long time ago. Dad's stationed in New Jersey, and Mom lives in Colorado. I have two brothers and a sister, and we've spent our lives bouncing back and forth between our parents. Don't get me wrong," he added hastily, "I love my folks. I just wish I could show you a snapshot—and have it be our original family unit." He stared at a blank wall a few feet away.

How would I feel if I were in Jon's place? Karen asked herself, and found the question almost impossible to comprehend. She realized that most of her security depended on her parents' close, loving support.

Of course as a Christian Karen knew that God was supposed to be her rock, her security. She had asked Christ to forgive her sins and come into her life when she was eleven. But she hadn't yet needed to depend on him for much more than assurance of her salvation. She was thankful that she hadn't yet had to face crises such as death, financial problems, serious illness, or any of a hundred other threatening situations. *The word that describes me,* she thought, *is "sheltered."*

Even so, she often felt insecure now that she was at college. Being away from home made her feel as though she were bouncing through life on an emotional and spiritual pogo stick. *I was never so moody before,* Karen realized. She found herself longing for the stability that her parents had provided.

Jon nudged her. "What are you thinking?" he asked. "I probably said more than I should have."

"No, of course not," she quickly reassured him. "By the way, are there any other Christians in your family?"

"Sure, my mom is. I don't think I'd be a Christian if it weren't for her." He grinned as he added, "I wouldn't be here studying for the ministry or talking to such a beautiful girl, either."

She laughed nervously and hoped that he hadn't noticed her blush.

"How about going out with me Friday night?" he asked. "I can get reservations at a fancy Italian place."

The silence seemed to stretch halfway to New York as Karen searched her jitterbugging brain for something to say. Finally she stammered, "I– I'd love to . . . b-b-b—"

"Great!" Jon answered enthusiastically. "I'll pick you up at seven!" He glanced at his watch. "I'm late for practice. Bye!" he shouted back over his shoulder as he took off for the gym.

"Wait!" Karen called weakly after him. "I wasn't finished," she muttered. *Now what will I do? I meant to tell him about Charles. I can't go—I'm engaged!* She frowned in confusion. *Didn't he notice the ring?* she wondered. The shimmering rock on her hand suddenly seemed to weigh a thousand pounds as she realized that she really did want to go out with Jon.

He fascinates me, she admitted as she tried to quell her guilty feelings about her relationship with Charles. *Who knows whether I'll ever have more than one date with Jon—but I do know this much: If I really loved Charles, then Jon never would have interested me.*

She sighed, realizing that she could no longer ignore the issue. *I have to talk to Charles right away—tonight,* she decided firmly. *I'm not being fair to him or me to let this go on any longer.* She stood up, suddenly feeling older and more responsible than she really wanted to be as she headed for the cafeteria.

The line of students snaked its way through several hallways and flights of stairs. Karen stood patiently at the end. It didn't matter—she wasn't hungry anyway.

"There you are!" Charles's voice intruded on her thoughts. "Where have you been?" he demanded. "I waited for you in the dorm for half an hour, and then I checked the music building, the library—"

She noticed that his hair and coat were soaked, and felt guiltier still. "I'm sorry, Charles. I guess I forgot what time it was," she apologized, hoping that he wouldn't question her further.

"It's OK. I was just concerned about you." He pointed at the line. "This will take forever. Want to go get a hamburger?"

"I'm not really hungry, but I'll go along for the ride." Karen's tone was unenthusiastic, for she knew that she couldn't avoid the subject of their engagement for long.

They dodged puddles in the downpour as they ran for the parking lot. Always the gentleman, Charles unlocked her car door first, rain streaming down the back of his neck. "Brrr!" he complained as he jumped in and started the motor.

They rode in silence for several miles. "You're sure quiet tonight," he commented as he turned down the volume on the radio. "Is something bugging you?"

"Yes." It was barely a whisper. She tried to

blink back the scalding tears, for she knew that he hated to see her cry.

"Well, let's talk about it right now." He glanced sharply at her and pulled to the side of the road. "Shoot. Take as long as you want—I'll listen." He settled back comfortably.

"I . . . I have a problem. No, we're the problem. . . ."

Charles sighed. "Go on, Karen," he prompted her as though he were indulging a troublesome child.

"I don't know how to say this right, but I don't want to marry you, Charles, because—" She stopped, unwilling to continue but knowing there was no turning back.

"Don't want to marry me? Why not?" He almost shouted the words.

Karen cringed. Charles was taking it far worse than she'd imagined. He was always so calm, so precise. She'd never seen him angry before.

Her words came out in a jumbled rush, "Because I don't love you—I mean I do—but just not in the right way." She bit her lip and stared down at her lap. She couldn't look at him—it hurt too much.

"What? I don't get it, Karen. What brought this on? Is there another guy?" His knuckles turned white as he gripped the steering wheel.

"No, not really. I've been wrong to let our relationship go on like this. I'm sorry, Charles. I know I'm hurting you, and I don't want to do that."

"You've told me from the beginning that you loved me, Karen. What's changed?"

"Nothing's changed." She swallowed her tears. "Everything's the same. It's just taken me this long to realize that we've never had that spark—that something extra that it takes to want to live with each other for the rest of our lives." She felt thoroughly frustrated as she glanced at Charles and saw his hurt, confused expression. *How else can I explain it?* she wondered, but tried again. "We don't have whatever it is that my parents have. After twenty-one years of marriage they still have a glow. We *never* had that, Charles."

"I think you're wrong. People express love in different ways. I *know* that I love you. That should be enough to satisfy you. The problem is that you and your family are just too emotional for your own good!" He sighed. "But I know I'll never convince you if that's the way you feel." He pocketed the ring that Karen handed him. "Let's go." He gunned the motor and headed back to the college.

Through her tears, Karen glanced over at him. His face seemed chiseled in granite. *What's he thinking?* she wondered. *I never know how he feels about anything. Charles just won't say.*

He drove up in front of Flanders Hall, and said stiffly, "I'd like my picture back, too."

She nodded and felt for the door handle since he made no move to open it for her. She jumped out and called back, "I'll get it now. Wait a minute."

She raced up to her room and grabbed his portrait off her desk, causing Tricia to stare wide-eyed at her. She slammed the door behind her and ran back downstairs. He was still waiting with the car motor running.

"Here, Charles." She thrust the picture at him and suddenly felt awkward. What could she say? And what about the weeks and months ahead? They'd be sure to bump into each other on campus.

"Karen," he said, and his voice sounded as though there was gravel in his throat. "Can I kiss you good-bye?"

Figuring it was the least she could do, she leaned forward. As he kissed her, she tasted tears, and felt as though she had only rubbed salt into the wounds she had inflicted on him.

"Bye, Charles," she whispered, as she slowly turned away. "I *am* sorry."

CHAPTER

2

KAREN woke early the next morning and ran to the window to open the drapes. To her delight, she saw that the sun was shining, reflected a million times in the rain-soaked grass and puddles. "Wake up, Trish!" she urged. "It's a beautiful day!"

Tricia sat up, stifling a yawn. "Is it that time already?" she groaned, and then burrowed back under the covers. Her head reappeared a moment later. "*You're* sure in a good mood!" she observed in an accusing tone.

Karen stared at her uncomprehendingly for a moment. Then it all came back to her—the scene with Charles the night before, and the bitter tears she'd shed afterward. No wonder Tricia seemed a little sarcastic at her sudden good spirits. Karen hardly knew how to answer her friend.

"I don't feel good about hurting Charles, if that's what you mean," she said slowly. "You know why I broke the engagement—it was the only honest thing I could do."

"I'm not arguing with that," Tricia broke in. "I just don't understand how you can bounce back so fast! I thought you'd be devastated for weeks."

Karen threw her hands up helplessly. "I don't know why, but the truth is, I *do* feel good today! I'm relieved, I guess, that the whole thing's over, but it's deeper than that. . . . Am I making any sense?"

Tricia's expression became thoughtful. "Yes," she agreed finally. "I think I understand. What you're really feeling is freedom—and you deserve that. But marriage shouldn't make people feel trapped. Maybe the key is to love the right person," she suggested. "Then you'd still feel free even if you *were* married. Now, does *that* make sense?"

Karen smiled. It felt good to be free.

During the following week, she looked forward to her date with Jon. Not that she had any intention of getting all tangled up in a relationship again. Still, it would be fun to go out with someone new and interesting.

The days seemed endless to Karen until Friday evening finally came. "I've never been this excited about a date," she confessed to Tricia as she tried on her third dress, a creamy white, peasant-style with lace trim.

"I can tell," Tricia remarked dryly and then giggled. "Why don't you wear your red dress? Then if you drop a spicy meatball, it won't show!" She grinned impishly.

"That's not funny! I don't have anything special to wear," Karen complained. "This dress shrank last time I washed it and now the sleeves are too short. What'll I wear?" she wailed.

"The dress you have on. It was good enough to wear to church last Sunday."

Karen tugged at the zipper on yet another outfit—the one that Tricia had originally suggested. "How does this look?" she asked as she critically examined her image in the mirror. The dark red, ultra-suede dress complemented her figure and porcelain complexion.

"You look chic—very Italian!" Tricia teased.

"I'm not trying to look Italian," Karen protested and started to take it off.

"Quit it!" Tricia shrieked. "I was joking! Now relax. What really counts is if Jon thinks you're special. Then he'll never notice what you're wearing anyway. You could model a flour sack!" She shoved Karen out the door. "Go on now. He's been waiting long enough in that crummy lobby."

Calm down—relax! Be cool. Take your time. . . . Karen pep-talked her emotions as she went to meet Jon. But then she saw him waiting for her, and her hard-won composure vanished as quickly as a magician's silk scarves. He seemed even more handsome than ever. His well-tailored denim suit gave him a suave, but casual look.

"Hi, Karen! You look terrific!" he said as he stepped forward to meet her. She could tell by his appreciative glance that he really meant the compliment, and she was glad she'd worn the red dress.

Jon led her to his car, a rather old Ford sedan. She noticed that it was freshly waxed and spotless inside and out as he held the door open for her. He switched on the radio and sang along as they headed down the freeway.

"You have a nice voice," she complimented him. "Do you sing in the choir?"

"No, basketball takes too much time, but I'd like to. I always sang in the church choir back home, and I miss it." He glanced at Karen. "How about you?"

"I'm taking oratorio this semester. I play the clarinet, too, and I'm thinking about signing up for band next year."

"Is that right?" Jon asked. "I'm in band—play a mean trombone. You ought to join. We could use another good clarinet player."

He pulled up to a place called "Angelo's." It seemed small but inviting. A stained-glass window graced the restaurant's entrance. As they entered, Karen thought she could hear a violinist playing faintly in the background. She sniffed delightedly at the enticing aroma that wafted toward them.

Jon seemed perfectly poised throughout the evening. Karen soon forgot that she'd ever been nervous as they found so much to talk about. They discovered that they both shared a love of Shakespeare's plays, and Jon promised to take her to a Saturday market.

"You'll like it, Karen," he said confidently.

"There are strolling musicians, jugglers, and all kinds of ethnic food. The atmosphere is incredible—almost like going back to the eighteenth century! There are rows of little booths where people make and sell candles, pottery, and just about anything you can imagine—right there in front of you!"

"You're right. I *would* enjoy that!" she agreed.

"How about the Space Needle? Have you been there yet? Or Underground Seattle? That's fascinating if you like history!"

Karen shook her head. "I haven't been anywhere other than a few movies and shopping centers—but I do like historical places. Museums fascinate me."

"Wow! Then I have a bundle of places to take you! Want to go?"

She laughed. "Of course I do. In what order?"

"How about starting with a Saturday market? We could go tomorrow morning right after breakfast." She nodded, overcome with surprise, but Jon didn't seem to notice. He glanced at his watch and signaled the waiter for the bill.

As they drove back to the college, Karen sneaked a few sideway glances at Jon's handsome profile. He seemed so different from anyone she'd ever met—so special in some unaccountable way. She wasn't sure why she was attracted to him, but she regretted that the evening had to end.

After he'd left her at the front door of Flanders Hall, she hurried up the stairs as fast as her high heels would let her. She was certain that Tricia would be anxiously waiting for an instant replay of the evening.

But she was fast asleep. "Hey, wake up!" Karen hissed to her slumbering roommate. "Trish," Karen tried again, "I have to talk to you!"

"Oh, Karen, let me sleep." She rolled over and began to snore raucously.

"That's a fake job if I ever heard one." Karen laughed as she pulled Tricia's foot from under the covers. "I guess I'll have to tickle you awake!" she threatened.

"Have mercy!" Tricia begged. "OK, I'll listen to you. Just let go of my foot!"

Long after she had detailed the important event and Tricia had yawned herself back to sleep, Karen lay awake savoring each moment of that perfect evening. . . .

The weeks passed quickly for Karen. December was filled with tree trims, caroling, the Christmas banquet, shopping trips, Handel's "Messiah"—all shared with Jon. She barely thought about the final exams that also accompanied the holiday season. "I'm having so much fun, I'm not sure I want to go home for Christmas!" she joked to Tricia as they sat on their beds wrapping presents.

"Whatever happened to your terminal case of homesickness?" Tricia asked. "Your parents are going to be mighty jealous of Jon when they find out what he's done."

"What's he done?"

"Why he's stolen your affections, dear girl! *That's* what he's done," Tricia teased, and then frowned darkly. "Who knows what they'll do to him when they find out!"

"Oh, don't worry. I won't tell them!"

"Got the tape over there?" Tricia asked as she plowed through mountains of gift wrap. "You won't have to tell them—they'll figure it out for themselves. All I hear these days is 'Jon, Jon, Jon,'" she mimicked in her highest soprano.

"I'm not that bad!"

"Oh, yes you are! Jon Hamilton seems to be the only subject you're studying these days. Too bad there's no final. You'd get an *A* for sure!"

But Karen didn't seem to notice Tricia's sarcasm as she stared dreamily out the window. *Jon is so special,* she told herself. *And I'm so lucky to be dating him. If only. . . .* She came back to earth as a pillow connected with her head.

Tricia grinned mischieviously. "Well! Who were you thinking about?"

"Bet you couldn't guess! You know what, Trish?"

"No, come to think of it—what?"

"I can't figure him out," Karen confessed with a sigh. "How many times has he taken me out?" She added them up. "Let's say at least fifteen times if you count jogging in the park."

Tricia waited impatiently. "Are we still on the same subject? What don't I know?"

Karen made a face. "Jon hasn't kissed me yet," she admitted glumly, "and there's plenty of mistletoe around if he needs an excuse. How come he hasn't?"

"Maybe you need to change your toothpaste. I

know the store brand's cheaper but—" She ducked the stuffed tiger that Karen sent flying her way.

"Think he's scared of me because I'm a pastor's daughter?"

"Naw, I don't think Jon Hamilton would be scared of anything, much less kissing you."

"I'm beginning to think he never will. . . . But why won't he?"

"Ask him," Tricia suggested, a note of irritation in her voice.

Karen glanced at the French provincial alarm clock on her nightstand. Charles had given it to her last Christmas. She wondered briefly how he was doing. "Gotta go," she told Tricia. "Jon's supposed to meet me at the library in ten minutes. I have to study for that American history final tomorrow. Bye."

"You mean you're leaving me with this mess?" Tricia pointed at the disaster area. Half-filled suitcases leaked clothing, ribbons and wrapping paper were strewn everywhere, and Styrofoam packing chips clung like parasites to the carpet and bedspreads. She picked vainly at a few. "If only we could trust the airlines not to annihilate our presents, we wouldn't have to put up with these pesky critters."

"Let's try newspaper next time," Karen suggested. "But don't worry, I'll be back in a couple of hours to help clean up. Bye!"

"I love him, I love him, I love him!" she sang under her breath as she bounced down the stairs and sprinted over to the library. She spotted Jon patiently waiting for her on a park bench.

"Hi, Karen. Ready to study?" he asked, reaching for her books.

"Never! But I suppose we'd better. I don't want to lose my scholarship, that's for sure!" They entered the library and chose a table in the far corner.

"I don't want to lose my basketball scholarship, either," Jon agreed. "Gotta keep up the grades *and* the jump shots. Who'd ever guess that basketball would finance studying for the ministry? But I'm not complaining. I really do love to play. Now if I can just keep those grades high enough—" He opened his French book with a flourish, propping it in front of him, and grinned at Karen. "I wouldn't have any problem if I had brains like yours," he teased.

She blushed. "Your brains are as good as mine. I have more time to study, that's all." But she found it hard to concentrate with Jon seated across the table from her. His head was bent intently over the textbook, making him unaware that she was studying *him. I love you!* she thought, and wished that it didn't have to be a secret.

Jon looked up at her curiously. "Are you done already?" he asked.

"No—I've just been thinking. . . ."

"About what?" he prompted her, laughing. When Karen didn't answer, he tried again. "What are you thinking about? Come on, tell me!"

"Oh, just that—" She hesitated for a second, and then impulsively blurted out, "I love you."

She blushed furiously and stared down at the polished oak library table in dismay as she realized what she'd just done. After what seemed a long time, she finally glanced up at him, hoping he'd answer that he loved her, too. But Jon said nothing. He just looked at her with a confused expression on his face.

"I'm sorry, Jon. I shouldn't have said that," she apologized, feeling thoroughly embarrassed. *He doesn't love me,* she told herself and almost immediately began to argue with her conclusion. *He does too love me—I know he feels the same way I do. I can tell by the way he acts and looks at me.* Then the little voice inside her argued back, *If he loves me, why wouldn't he say so?*

"Karen, I don't know how to say this because I don't want to hurt you." Jon paused and looked helplessly at her. "I think I love you," he explained, "but until I'm absolutely certain, I won't say that I do. I don't want to tell you something like that lightly. I want it to be genuine and lasting." He reached for her hand and squeezed it. "I'm not saying I don't love you.... Do you understand?"

She nodded and opened her history textbook without further comment. She tried to study but the words swam before her eyes. *I've blown it,* she thought, miserably aware that subtlety wasn't one of her outstanding virtues.

"Karen, do you want to go for a ride?" Jon asked suddenly. "We can come back later to study." He smiled at her as if nothing had happened. "I need some fresh air. This place stifles my brain cells!"

They gathered their books and headed for the parking lot. Jon didn't say anything as they drove along the highway. He seemed to be concentrating deeply—on what, Karen wished she knew. She tried to guess where they were going, and then as she noticed familiar landmarks, she knew that Jon had chosen her favorite park. She liked it because it had long, winding dirt paths to follow—none of that city asphalt or concrete. It was quiet, too.

Hand-in-hand, they climbed one of the hills overlooking the city. "Look at the lights, Jon!" she exclaimed.

"They are beautiful," he agreed and then quietly noted, "Your eyes are like that, too, Karen. Sometimes they just sparkle and shine—especially when you're happy and excited." He put his arm around her shoulder and she snuggled a little closer.

"I'm happy right now," she whispered, and then he bent his head and kissed her—not a short, sweet first-date kiss, but a gentle, lingering one.

"I'll miss you, Karen," he said, holding her tight. "I wish I could be with you during Christmas. It'll be a long three weeks."

"It'll go faster than you think. But I'll miss you too," she confessed. "By the way, I'm curious about something."

"What? Ask me anything," he answered with mock gallantry.

"Why did it take you so long to kiss me?"

Jon reddened, and then his eyes began to twinkle. "The truth is, I didn't want to risk getting turned down—but I enjoyed it so much that I'm sorry I waited so long." He leaned down and kissed her again.

"I suppose we'd better go back." Karen murmured reluctantly. She *had* to make *A*'s on her final exams and term papers. Her scholarship depended on it. *I should have been studying,* she scolded herself. *But I wouldn't have missed this for anything!*

CHAPTER

3

KAREN grabbed her belongings and waited impatiently at the exit door as the train chugged to a halt. She jumped lightly to the ground and hurried into the station. Where was Jon? She couldn't wait to see him! Christmas vacation had been entirely too long without him.

A moment later she was enveloped in his strong arms. "You know what, Karen?" Jon said between kisses. "I discovered something while you were away."

"What? Tell me! I can't stand the suspense!"

"I discovered ... that I love you!" He swung her up into the air.

"Hey, put me down! Are you absolutely sure?"

"Of course I'm sure. I told you that I wouldn't say it until I was positive." He kissed her again. "Karen, I do love you—will you be my steady girl?"

"Oh, yes," she whispered, "because I love you, too."

From then on, they spent every possible minute together—meals, moments between classes, college chapel services, jogging around campus, and study time in the library. Though they occasionally double-dated with Jon's roommates, Brad and Mike, and their girl friends, they preferred single-dating. "It's more fun just getting to know *you*!" Karen declared to Jon.

Their relationship deepened quickly as each day they discovered more and more about each other. They talked about their future together and outlined the goals they wanted to reach. Number one, they decided, had to be God. Their Christian growth was important, and Christ had to be the center of their relationship.

They chose to attend a church near the campus, and decided to involve themselves in the activities. Before long, they were singing in the choir and leading a children's club. "I really like our Sunday school class," Karen told Jon. "Especially Larry and Janie—they're super!"

"Yeah," he agreed. "They seem like people you could really count on. I'd like to get to know them better."

The weeks rushed by as Jon and Karen's courtship continued. "Look, Trish!" Karen exclaimed one early spring afternoon as she burst into their room. "Jon left this bouquet of daisies in my mailbox. Isn't he sweet?"

"Wow! Candy bars, love notes, poems, records, and now flowers! What's next? I will say, he sure does treat you right," Tricia observed.

"I know, and I don't deserve it. But I love it anyway!"

"I've noticed." Tricia yawned as she turned back to her schoolwork. "Excuse me, but I've got to get busy on this calculus assignment. Oh, are you aware that our biology term papers are due Friday?"

"They are? Oops! I guess I'd better get busy." Karen flopped on her bed. How had she missed that assignment? It must have been the day she and Jon skipped class to—she stopped as she uncomfortably remembered that day.

Jon had told her that he needed to study for a French quiz. "I'm afraid I'm going to flunk that class," he said. "I haven't been studying as much as I should."

"I'll help you. French is easy for me," Karen offered. "I'll just skip biology today. I hate that class anyhow. Professor Campbell is such a bore!"

Since the weather was sunny, they quickly decided to study at their favorite park. When they arrived, they found it deserted. They spread a picnic blanket on the grassy hillside and ate their hamburgers and milkshakes. Afterward, Jon lay back on the blanket and closed his eyes against the sun's glare.

"That's not studying," she teased him. She couldn't resist the perfect opportunity and leaned over to kiss him. Then he put his arms around her and pulled her down beside him. *We shouldn't be doing this,* she told herself sternly. *But it feels so natural, so comfortable. Besides, I can trust Jon not to go too far.* She felt that strange stirring deep in the pit of her stomach again—Jon called it "getting turned on." What-

35

ever it was, it sure felt good, she admitted.

"We're not doing much studying for your French quiz," she pointed out when they came up for air.

"We will—right now. Help me conjugate 'to love.'"

Karen giggled. "In French or English?"

"In English." He gently pushed her down on the blanket and leaned over her, kissing her insistently.

I should stop this, Karen thought wildly, but then decided that matters were still under control. She eagerly responded to his kisses and caresses until she suddenly felt his body slide over onto hers. Her eyes widened in surprise and he stopped immediately.

"We've gone too far—I'm sorry, Karen. I don't know what came over me, but I was wrong." He hung his head dejectedly. "Will you forgive me?"

"I'm sorry, too, Jon." Karen was near tears. "It was just as much my fault as it was yours. I'll forgive you if you'll forgive me."

"All right. But I think we'd better pray about this right now." He reached for her hand and squeezed it tightly as they bowed their heads. "Lord, we're sorry that we let our feelings get out of control. We didn't mean to, but you know how much we love each other. Please take complete charge of our lives and help us to do your will."

"And Lord," Karen added, "I feel so awful right now. Please forgive us both and give us strength—your strength—because I don't think we have enough of our own. Amen."

She looked up at Jon. "I feel better now," she told him. "I'm sure that God will help us. We can handle it!"

"I wish I were as sure," he answered slowly. "What we did really scared me. It wouldn't have taken too much more—"

"I know." *What if it* had *happened?* she asked herself, terrified at the thought.

"Karen, I don't want to ever do anything to hurt you. I love you too much."

"I love you, too, Jon, and I don't want to hurt you, either." She shivered and he pulled the picnic blanket over her shoulders. All the warmth and light had gone from the afternoon.

And Jon had flunked the quiz the next day, Karen remembered miserably. Worse yet, they still weren't doing too well at controlling the amount of time they spent alone kissing.

"Where are you and Jon going tonight?" Tricia asked, breaking into her thoughts. Getting a non-committal shrug from Karen, she continued in a hurt tone, "I feel as though I'm sharing a room with a stranger. You never seem to have time to talk or go shopping like we used to."

Karen didn't answer, but Tricia's remark stung. She felt guilty, and then quickly became irritated. *It's none of her business,* she thought defensively.

Jon and Karen now had time only for each other. They soon became tempted to skip student activities such as baseball games, hayrides, concerts, and picnics. It all seemed childish and boring compared with being alone together.

The more time they spent together, the more

intimate they became in every area of their lives. It wasn't long until their sexual attraction for each other became the main focus of their hours together. Neither of them knew much about sex, and most of their knowledge was actually misinformation.

Karen recalled the short talk that her mother had given to her. She'd been a fourth-grader then, and her mother had seemed more embarrassed than anything else. The subjects of menstruation and intercourse were covered, but Karen only felt confused and frightened about the facts she'd learned.

Intercourse, she was sure, had to be a totally revolting, painful experience. And when could a woman become pregnant? Karen tried to remember. She thought perhaps it happened each time the couple had intercourse. No, that couldn't be right, she realized. She remembered it had something to do with the menstrual cycle. It must be either right after or right before that you could get pregnant, she decided.

Before she and Jon had become so involved, she had believed that kissing and sexual intercourse were non-related activities. She couldn't imagine that she would ever be tempted to have sex before she was married. *But what is "sex," anyway?* she asked herself. *Where should we draw the line?*

She remembered being upset back in high school when a schoolmate had become pregnant. "What if that happened to me?" she had asked her mother.

"As long as you're a Christian and a good girl,

Karen, you have nothing to worry about," her mother had replied soothingly.

Ha! Karen thought. The fireworks of romance had already exploded that naive myth, shattering it in short order. She had plenty to worry about, though she felt she *was* trying to be a Christian as well as a "good girl." *It's just that love complicates things,* she told herself.

She and Jon had already found that the nebulous term "going too far" had no absolute line. The more passionate their kissing, the more inadequate it seemed as an expression of their love. It became harder all the time to keep their hands off each other.

I finally know what "petting" means, Karen reflected. *The old definition that "necking is from the neck up" and "petting is from the neck down" leaves a little bit to be desired. And nobody ever told me that it felt so good either—just that it was wrong.*

Even so, she and Jon were confident that they could stop "before it was too late." After all, they had asked God to protect and help them, hadn't they? However, "too late" happened faster than Jon and Karen had ever imagined possible.

How did we get so far out of control? Karen asked herself, still dizzy from the sudden turn of events. *Why didn't we stop in time?* The questions continued to race through her mind. She shivered in the cold night air and glanced anxiously around the immediate vicinity of the park. *I'd die if someone saw us,* she thought.

It was beautiful though, she told herself, and it didn't hurt that much. She tugged at her clothes, trying to properly arrange them as she wondered what Jon was thinking.

"Are you OK?" he asked. "Do you feel bad about what we did? You know. . . ." He looked uncomfortable.

Karen frowned as she tried to understand his question. "Do you mean the fact that I'm not a virgin anymore?" she asked. "Why? Does it matter to you?"

"Well, of course it matters! What do you think I am? I still love you and I always will. But it makes me feel bad that I took something like that away from you—"

"You didn't take it away, Jon. I *gave* it—and I love you. I didn't really expect that to happen, but it's too late to change things."

Jon shook his head. "We didn't do anything different this time than we did any other time—kissing, petting and all—but this time we just didn't stop in time."

Although Karen had enjoyed the initial experience of intercourse, she was beginning to feel guilty. *I'm not a virgin anymore,* kept running through her thoughts. *Does it matter?* she asked herself. *Will it matter the rest of my life?*

She suddenly remembered a warning her father had given her years before when she'd gone steady with her first boyfriend. "Karen, if you ever got pregnant out of wedlock, I'd have to leave the ministry. I couldn't hold my head up and preach to others if I couldn't control my own child," he'd told her sternly. It was the only time she'd ever heard him mention the subject of sex. His words had frightened her then. Now she was terrified at the possibility of causing hurt and pain to her parents.

"Jon, what if I got pregnant because of tonight?" She told him what her father had said. "And Jon, you'd never have the chance to be a minister, either, and that's what God has called you to do. Besides that, we'd both be expelled from Wellington—wouldn't *that* look good on our transcripts!"

"Yeah, and my dad said he'd disown me if I ever got a girl pregnant." He buried his head in his hands. "I've gotten us into a fine mess!"

"It's just as much my fault," she pointed out. As she pondered their problem, the answer seemed obvious. "Jon, we'll just have to stop—everything. There's no other solution."

"But I don't want to quit seeing you," he disagreed. "I love you too much. But you're right. We can't run these risks any longer."

"I don't want to stop seeing you, either. But every time we're together it gets worse! If we couldn't stop ourselves before, then what makes us think we can in the future?" She saw that his expression was stubborn. *He's not about to give up our relationship,* Karen realized, *and I don't want to, either. I love him too much. But what are we going to do?*

"Why don't we get married?" he suggested.

His spur-of-the-moment proposal shocked Karen. She shook her head. "I'd be thrilled to be engaged to you, but you know we aren't ready for marriage. For one thing," she pointed out, "we're broke. Neither of us has a cent in savings. It all goes for tuition."

"You're right. I wanted to wait until graduation to marry you. From a financial standpoint, it won't work any other way. But that's a whole year from now." He frowned, and she could tell that something else was on his mind. "What about using a contraceptive?" he suggested finally. "Wouldn't that solve the problem—just in case?"

She thought hard about that one. "No, Jon. That would be the same as planning to have sex, and I feel guilty enough about it just happening. And besides, I'd be too embarrassed to buy the stuff. What if someone I knew saw me? Or what if Tricia found it?" She shuddered.

"It isn't much of an answer, is it?" he agreed. "We'll just have to quit. It won't be easy, but we can do it."

But how? Karen wondered silently. She knew God had promised to help them overcome temptation, but she realized that lately they'd neglected to ask for his aid. In fact, she admitted, the few times they had stopped to pray, they'd practically asked for his blessing.

She felt ashamed as she remembered praying, "Lord, we really do want to honor you and do your will in our lives. Thank you for bringing us together and for giving us love to express. Please guide our time together." And then what followed could have been part of an R-rated movie. How mixed up could they get? she asked herself in disgust as she resolved to change the course of their relationship.

But in the weeks that followed, Karen found that it wasn't so simple to carry out her good intentions. She and Jon tried to control themselves, but it seldom worked. Their sexual relationship controlled them instead.

"What are we going to do?" Karen cried in frustration. "What if we get caught? What if I get pregnant? Jon, I'm really afraid! My period's late again and I feel nauseated. What if I *am* pregnant?"

"What? I thought you were paying attention to the right and wrong days—you know what I mean!—when it's safe and when it's not!"

"I have been! Don't yell at me!"

"Don't cry, Karen. I'm sorry." He patted her shoulder awkwardly. "Maybe we should go see Dr. Miller. He could give you a test to find out. There's no sense worrying about something if it's not even true."

"But I don't want to go see *him*. He knows us!"

"I think we can trust him. Dr. Miller has always been easy to talk to, and we really do need to get some answers." He waited for her decision.

Karen felt trapped. She didn't want anyone to know what they were doing—much less a doctor who provided the health care for the entire college. But Jon was right. Dr. Miller seemed to be a compassionate person. "All right," she agreed finally. "I'll go if you'll go with me."

"Fine. I'll set up the appointment."

Later, as they sat waiting in the doctor's office, Karen wished that she could run away from the whole situation. "Did you tell the nurse why you were making the appointment?" she asked.

"Nope." Jon didn't have much to say that day.

After what seemed to be a long wait, Dr. Miller ushered them both into his office. "Now what can I do for you today?" he asked as they nervously took the chairs he offered.

I'll bet he already knows, Karen thought to herself. *What else do a frightened-looking couple have on their minds?* She tried to answer, but the words froze in her throat. She gave Jon a mute plea as tears filled her eyes.

"We're afraid that Karen's pregnant," Jon answered finally.

Dr. Miller nodded understandingly. "Do you remember which days you had intercourse?" he asked. Karen blushed as she handed him her calendar showing the days of her menstrual cycle. She pointed out to him the times she and Jon had had sex.

The doctor studied the calendar while Karen fidgeted. "Well, except for the times during the middle of your cycle, you are probably safe," he informed them.

"The *middle*?" Karen squeaked in dismay. "I thought it was either right before or right after my period that I could get pregnant."

"You've got your information backwards, Karen. Have you been using any type of birth control?" He looked questioningly at each of them, but they shook their heads.

"Well, if you're going to keep this up and you don't want to end up pregnant you're going to have to use it," Dr. Miller told them bluntly.

"Why?" Karen asked. "I don't want anymore to do with sex, and Jon doesn't either. We've talked about it and we've decided that it's not right. We *have* to stop."

Dr. Miller shook his head. "You're not alone," he said. "Many couples have gotten into the habit of having sex, and then later decided to quit. But it's not that easy. Once you begin, it's next to impossible to stop. Let me prescribe a birth control pill, Karen," he suggested. "It's the easiest method with the lowest failure rate."

"No thanks, Doctor," she refused firmly. "We can stop—if it's not already too late."

"All right. I can't force you to use a contraceptive, but I wish you'd listen."

He turned to Jon. "A condom would be a solution that *you* could responsibly use, and you can buy it in any drugstore, no questions asked." Jon acknowledged Dr. Miller's suggestion with a silent nod.

"You can wait for Karen in the lobby, Jon," the doctor said, dismissing him.

Then he called his nurse in to give Karen a shot. "If you're pregnant," he explained, "this shot will prevent the egg from attaching to the lining of the uterus. You can telephone about the test results in a few days. Keep your chin up!" He smiled encouragingly as he left the room.

"The doctor will only prescribe this shot once," the nurse warned Karen. "After that, you take the consequences. And by the way, this isn't foolproof."

Great, Karen thought. *Just what I wanted to hear*.

She felt edgy for the next few days, as though

she were standing in the jaws of a huge trap and wondering if she'd already tripped the spring. Finally the waiting was over, and she ran to tell Jon. "The test was negative! I'm not pregnant!" He held her tightly and they both cried tears of relief. *At least we learned our lesson in time*, she thought.

CHAPTER

4

"HERE'S your mail, Karen," Tricia said as she entered their room. "I thought I'd save you the trip. How's the studying coming along?"

"Oh, Trish—how did I ever get so far behind? I haven't even read some of this stuff yet!" Karen gestured at the foot-high pile of books on her desk.

"How *did* you get so far behind?" Tricia mocked. Then she apologized, "Sorry, I'll save the lectures. Maybe I'll need them when I fall in love." She sighed dramatically and rolled her eyes. "When, when, *when?*"

Karen shuffled through the assortment of mail. "Spiritual Life Retreat—what's that?"

"Where have you been? That's all anybody's been talking about for weeks. You and Jon are going, aren't you?"

"Probably." Karen scanned the flyer for information. "A weekend in the woods does sound

47

terrific. But what's the speaker going to talk about? Isn't it sort of unusual to have a medical doctor?"

"I think he might be a psychologist," Tricia guessed. "I hadn't thought much about it, but I'm sure he'll be good. Everybody says the retreat is the highlight of the year."

"I'll probably need a retreat just to recuperate from midterms. I may need a doctor, too!" Karen giggled as she opened another textbook. "Right now, though, I'd better get my mind on the anatomy of a frog or I'll flunk biology."

"Ribit, ribit!" Tricia croaked encouragingly.

Karen's midterm results were mostly C's, but she shrugged off her poor performance. *I'll make it up on the finals and term papers,* she told herself. She pushed the subject of grades to the bottom of her list. There wasn't room at the top, for Jon had taken first priority months ago.

His grades were suffering, too, especially French. Karen had offered to drill him on vocabulary and verb tenses, but the sessions never lasted long. They both preferred kissing to studying.

The following weekend the entire college packed up and headed to the wilderness for the annual retreat. For the first time in a long while, Karen found herself becoming excited about something other than Jon. Of course, if he hadn't attended, she wouldn't have gone, either.

Karen sensed that both of them needed spiritual help. *Maybe Jon and I will get straightened out here,* she thought hopefully as they pulled up to the main lodge. She had to admit she felt far from God, and she wondered uncomfortably if her relationship with Jon could be the reason. They hadn't stuck by their decision to stop having sex. If anything, they'd become more involved. Sex *was* a problem, but they just didn't seem to know what to do about it.

She doubted, though, that they would find help for *that* problem at the retreat, for she believed that she and Jon were alone in their dilemma. Karen didn't think any other couples at Wellington Christian College were tempted by premarital sexual involvement.

But even if that premise were true, Dr. Larson must have disagreed, for his topic was "sex" during each session for three solid days—much to Karen's chagrin! She felt that he was preaching straight at her each time. Every session she insisted that she and Jon sit as far back as possible. Their secret tormented her relentlessly as the doctor hammered away at the formerly taboo subject.

"Men, I want to address myself to you," Dr. Larson announced. Karen's mind snapped to attention. *What will he say to* them? she wondered.

"Women have always received all the lectures and responsibility in the area of sex, and it's an unfair double standard," he declared emphatically. "I want you fellows to be aware that women are not like pop bottles." The audience stirred noisily as the last few drowsing brains on automatic pilot switched over and began receiving data. Pop bottles? What did they have in common with women?

Dr. Larson grinned as he noted the students' complete attention. Then his expression became serious as he explained his illustration. "You see, men, you can take a bottle back to the store after you've used it, and get a refund. Or if it's no deposit, no return, you can toss it into the nearest garbage can—shattering it into a million pieces if you like. But a woman is not a thing." He paused to let that profound fact soak in.

"You'd better treat her like a fragile, priceless vase, because you have your life invested—and so does she," he pointed out. "You see, you've both made a deposit, and there's no return in God's book. Once you've begun a sexual relationship, you belong to each other. And if you begin that relationship before marriage, you stand responsible to God for the consequences."

Dr. Larson continued, but Karen's mind was back on the pop bottles. *I wonder if Jon would ever be tempted to "return me to the store" for someone new?* she worried. She felt that she would never want to marry anyone else if she and Jon broke off their relationship. But no, that wouldn't happen, she thought, trying to reassure herself. She and Jon loved each other far too much. They were as good as married in her mind. Still—she glanced apprehensively at him, and reached over to grasp his hand. He squeezed hers, and then she felt secure.

After Dr. Larson finished speaking, he opened the floor to questions from students. Karen was amazed at the blunt inquiries voiced by her classmates: "What is oral sex? Is it wrong?"

"When is a woman most likely to become pregnant?" "Do women climax?" "What if a couple goes all the way? Can they stop having sex and still go together?" "Will it physically or emotionally hurt a man if he's 'turned on' and the couple does not have complete intercourse?"

Karen was too shocked and embarrassed to cope with such a frank discussion of intimate matters, so she left the meeting early. Jon, however, stayed to hear all the details. It was small comfort to Karen that most of the students seemed as confused and ignorant as she and Jon were.

Alone in her cabin, she agonized over the fact that she wanted answers, but yet she didn't want them. Her ignorance had blanketed her actions in the recent past, and she feared that knowing the facts might be too penetrating and uncomfortable. Nevertheless, she mistrusted the old saying, "What you don't know won't hurt you." She had discovered that what she didn't know *could* sometimes prove quite painful.

The next morning, Karen was sitting under a tree trying vainly to meditate and pray when Charles approached her. "Hi, Karen. I've been wanting to talk to you. Can I sit down?"

"Sure. How've you been?"

"Fine." He sat on a large boulder next to her as she looked at him curiously. But Charles didn't seem eager to begin the conversation. Instead, he seemed intent on inspecting the pine needles and bugs on the ground.

For wanting to talk to me, he's not saying

very much, she thought uneasily. "What's on your mind?" she prompted him.

"I don't know exactly how to say this to you. . . ." He stopped and scratched his head in frustration.

Karen waited patiently. She suddenly felt that she might not care for whatever it was that Charles wanted to say.

"I . . . I'm concerned about you, Karen," he began hesitantly. "I still care about you very much."

"I care about you, too, Charles. My decision hasn't changed, though."

He shook his head. "That's not what I'm getting at. I know it's all over between us." He looked helplessly at her for a long moment and then said in a choked voice, "People are talking about you and Jon. Some of the guys have said that you two are really heavy into making out. . . ."

"That's ridiculous!" Karen retorted. "I can't believe that you'd listen to gossip like that!"

"I don't want to believe it, Karen, but I can tell just by looking at Jon that he's a—a wolf! Please get away from him before it's too late!"

"That's not true, Charles! Jon is *not* any such thing! You have an overactive imagination and you're just jealous." She was near tears. But not wanting to give him the satisfaction she willed herself not to cry.

Charles sighed. "I'm not jealous, Karen. I just don't want to see you hurt. If you say it's not true, then I believe you and I'm glad. But I don't

trust Jon, and I hope you'll be careful, that's all."
He looked uncomfortably at her. "I guess I'd better head for breakfast. See you later," he said and
waved good-bye.

She stared wordlessly after him, afraid that he
knew the awful truth and wasn't a bit fooled by
her lies. *And I've never been a liar before now,*
she thought, sick at how covering up one sin
had led to another. *But Jon's not a wolf!* she argued. *Everything that's happened is my fault
too—and it's a result of our human weakness.
Charles acted like Jon was ready to destroy me,
but I know Jon loves me.* She clung desperately
to that fact as she wondered how Charles had
come across his information.

But she soon forgot about the disturbing conversation as the retreat activities filled up most
of her time. The weekend passed quickly, and
Jon and Karen scarcely had time to talk to each
other.

A wilderness hike was scheduled on the last
afternoon, and Karen wanted to go with Jon.
Where is he? she wondered as she searched the
grounds several times. As the dinner bell rang,
she finally located him. "Where were you?" she
asked. "I was worried about you!" She was also a
bit angry that he hadn't included her in his plans
or at least told her what he intended to do.

"I'll tell you later," Jon replied nervously,
glancing at the students around them. They carefully balanced their trays as they walked to a table on the far side of the room. That way they
could talk undisturbed for a while until the ta-

bles closer to the cafeteria line were filled. It also signaled to others that they wanted to be alone—as usual.

"Well, where did you go?" Karen asked him again as they sat down.

"If you *must* know, I had an appointment with the speaker," Jon answered in an irritated manner. "Now can I eat?"

"No! Not until you tell me what you talked about!"

"I told him about us and asked for advice. That's all." Jon munched on his fried chicken as Karen tried to swallow the news that their relationship wasn't a secret to Dr. Larson.

That's just great! she thought sarcastically. *Way to blow it, Jon Hamilton!* It unnerved her that he would actually tell someone what they were involved in. It was bad enough that Dr. Miller knew their secret. What if Dr. Larson told the dean or the president of the college? Karen felt betrayed.

With difficulty she managed to squelch all the "what if's" that were churning around her. "What did he say?" she asked.

"He asked me to write him a letter in three years to let him know how our lives turn out. He said he couldn't prophesy a successful marriage under the circumstances."

"But, Jon, we love each other! We're going to get married as soon as we can. What could happen to that?" Dr. Larson's note of doom angered her. She sat silently, watching Jon devour both his food and her untouched meal. How could he eat in the middle of such a crisis? "Do you be-

54

lieve what he said about us?" she asked, hoping he'd answer no.

"I don't know, Karen. What he said makes sense, but I do know that I love you and want to marry you. We'll work it out somehow. Now stop worrying so much." He polished off her piece of banana cream pie and then stood up. "Is your luggage ready?" he asked. "We'd better start back right away. I have a seven-thirty class in the morning."

"Don't remind me," Karen groaned. She felt depressed at the thought of textbooks, term papers, and grades. It was strange how her attitude toward school had changed, she realized in a flash of insight. In the past, learning had always been a game. She'd even been the valedictorian of her high school graduating class. Now her accomplishments seemed to be ancient history, especially when she was faced with present reality. She could hardly believe that she, Karen Blackburn, could have received *C*'s on her midterms!

Jon had fared even worse. He received a warning note as a result of his midterm French exam. If he didn't improve that *D* grade, he'd be on probation. His next year's basketball scholarship could be jeopardized.

But however poor their scholastic records had become, Jon and Karen's romance flourished. It didn't seem as though Dr. Larson's dismal prediction had any chance of coming true, for the only cloud on the horizon was their impending summer separation.

They discussed it at length, and decided that the separation would be a good endurance test of their love. If they still felt the same way about each other in the fall, they planned to announce their engagement.

A few days before spring term ended, Karen received an official letter from the school. "Jon, look at this! What am I going to do?" she cried. "It's from the dean. He says that I've lost my scholarship! That's not fair!" she raged bitterly. "I still have an *A-* average, and I took some upper division classes. That should count for something!"

Jon also found bad news in his mailbox. "Oh, no!" he groaned. "I have to repeat last term's French class in order to graduate next year—and that'll cost extra tuition money." He sighed. "I guess I don't have much choice, do I? At least I didn't lose my basketball scholarship—yet." His face was glum.

Karen made an appointment to see the dean. But when she expressed her arguments about the school's decision to him, he disagreed. "I'm sorry, Karen. The competition's a lot tougher in college. You received your academic scholarship because you were a high school valedictorian. But in order to maintain it, your grade point average would have had to be much higher. Several freshmen maintained straight *A*'s," he pointed out. "Unfortunately, you weren't one of them. However, I'll do what I can. Perhaps we can give you a music scholarship. I see here on your transcript that you were in your high school marching band."

She nodded. "I plan to audition tomorrow," she said meekly.

"Don't worry too much," he consoled her. "We want you to return to Wellington next year. Perhaps we can increase your loan. You are a good student, though I think you're capable of doing better than this year's record indicates." He smiled encouragingly as he dismissed her.

Jon was waiting outside the office for her. They walked silently through the campus mall. "This whole business is completely unfair!" Karen suddenly exploded. "Why should I *have* to play a clarinet in order to go to school? What if I don't *want* to?"

"No, Karen," Jon gently disagreed. "It's fair. You know that the teachers and the scholarship committee acted on the facts. The truth is, we've been unfair to ourselves and our future—and now we're paying for it."

In her heart, Karen knew Jon was right. But it's still unfair, she stubbornly insisted as she worried about how she would pay for her sophomore year of college. The music scholarship wasn't a sure thing, and she hated the idea of increasing her loan.

Worst of all, she could see more storm clouds gathering ahead. *What will I tell Mom and Dad?* she wondered.

"IT'S so good to be home again!" Karen told her parents as they exchanged hugs and kisses. She felt grateful to be surrounded by the security of her home, church, and small town. But much to her dismay, she soon discovered that nothing was exactly the way she'd left it a year ago. She knew she had changed, but she hadn't realized that her parents would seem different, too. Her relationship with them was frequently strained.

After a year of freedom and decision-making, she was once again under their authority, subject to their rules and opinions. She had almost forgotten what it was like to be told where she could or could not go, what she should wear, and what time she was expected home.

Karen's college grades were also a matter of contention between them. Her parents had received a letter about the scholarship she'd lost—no matter that it had been replaced by a music scholarship of equal value. They wanted to know why her grades had slipped. *If they only knew,* Karen thought guiltily, but then shifted to a defensive attitude. *If they didn't always pressure me so much. . . .*

Karen had always tried to be obedient and to make her parents proud of her. They continually challenged her to do her best—and then to go one step beyond. *What is my best?* Karen often thought in frustration. *No matter how hard I try, it's never enough!*

Her parents also expected her to be an example to the church and community. She often resented the "goody-goody" image that her friends teased her about—not that she particularly wanted to do bad things. She was just tired of people expecting her to be perfect, especially when she knew she wasn't.

Then, too, in her year away at college, she realized that when she made decisions that didn't reflect her parents' choices, she didn't sense condemnation from God or others—she only felt guilty about how her parents would react.

Of course, that didn't apply to her relationship with Jon. Karen knew that no one would approve of some of her decisions in that area. Even so, she felt that their love for each other was genuine. She was sure that God meant for them to be married. She thought about him constantly. She remembered his smile, his laugh, his sensitive nature, his predictable habits, his walk. How could she have been lucky enough for him to choose her?

Karen's relationship with Jon was the biggest

issue that she faced with her parents. Though they had never met him, she sensed their disapproval of him, and she didn't understand why. *Maybe it's just my imagination,* she thought, *because I feel guilty about what's been going on and I know they'd be upset if they knew. No, "upset" isn't the word for it—"shattered" is more like it.*

It wasn't that her parents had ever said anything against him. But Karen noticed, or *thought* she noticed, a hesitation from them whenever she mentioned him. She had no concrete evidence that they didn't like him, but she had an uneasy feeling that wouldn't leave.

I'm probably overreacting and being defensive, she admitted. *Maybe it's because of Charles.* She was glad that he'd stayed in Seattle to work instead of coming home, too. He'd only complicate matters and set the tongues to wagging, she figured. She supposed that breaking her engagement with him and then immediately becoming seriously involved with Jon probably made her parents worried.

One morning, Karen and her mother were relaxing over cups of coffee. Karen bubbled on and on about Jon. "And we plan to announce our engagement in September," she said impulsively, glancing at her mother. To her dismay, Mom looked displeased, her mouth set in a tight, thin line.

"I've been wanting to talk with you about something for quite awhile, Karen," she said. "I guess now is as good a time as any."

"What's on your mind?" Karen felt uneasy.

61

"It seems to me that I hear the name 'Jon' in every sentence," her mother noted, a slight frown creasing her forehead.

"I can't help it, Mom. I miss him so much! Can't you remember when you and Dad first fell in love?"

"Yes, I remember. But you're so young, Karen. Your father and I hoped that you would finish college first, and then think about marriage."

"But you and Dad were only nineteen when you got married," Karen argued. "It worked out just fine!" She knew she'd cornered her mother there.

But her mother wasn't beaten that easily. "Yes," she countered, "but I've always regretted that I didn't finish college. I've never again had the opportunity, and I don't have near the talent and brains that you've been blessed with. I'd hate to see you waste them."

Now Karen was angry. "Do you call marriage and a family *wasting* talent and brains?" she stormed. "For your information, that's all I've ever really wanted! I don't care about a big education. I just want to be happy—but I always have to live up to *your* expectations!"

While Karen sobbed, her mother sat silently watching her. There were tears in her eyes, too. "Karen," she said finally, "I want you to be happy. Really, I do. We just aren't sure that Jon is the right person for you.

"And do you know why we feel that way?" she continued. "Because you're so different from the Karen we've always known. You constantly tell us how great Jon is and how well he does everything. Then you run yourself and your own accomplishments down. We can't understand this. If Jon is truly supposed to be your mate, then he should enhance your qualities, not detract from them."

"But he does!" Karen argued. "I guess I keep telling you about him because I want you to like him. You don't even know him and already you're making unfair judgments. Mom," she pleaded, "give Jon a decent chance. Please?"

Her mother nodded her head and seemed about to continue the conversation when the telephone rang. As she went to answer it, Karen thankfully escaped.

In the weeks that followed, she found it difficult, if not impossible, to talk to her mother. A heavy curtain of silence hung between them. Karen spent as much time as possible out of the house. When she wasn't working as a waitress at the Country Kettle, she walked for hours on the beach, built intricate sand castles, and wrote letters to Jon.

Though she wrote nearly every day, she was lucky to hear from him once every other week. His last letter had contained some exciting news—he was coming to visit on August twenty-fifth. He planned to stay for a week, then they'd drive back together to Seattle to start school.

She wondered what kind of a reception her parents would give him. They had so many old-fashioned ideas, one of which concerned engagement protocol. They would expect Jon to *ask* for the privilege of marrying her, and they wouldn't give their permission until they were certain he was the best qualified husband for her.

Though Karen didn't need their permission to legally marry, she was reluctant to go against their wishes. *But Jon is the one I love,* she thought defensively, *and they're just going to have to accept him.*

The days crawled by as she planned for Jon's arrival. She was glad that he was coming during the county fair—he'd enjoy that! Her friends had planned a beach party in his honor, too. *We'll have plenty to do,* she thought happily.

When she felt she couldn't stand the anticipation another minute, Jon finally arrived. He was as charming as ever, but it didn't work on Karen's mother, who regarded him with ill-concealed suspicion. *This isn't going to be easy,* Karen thought, disappointed and discouraged. *Mom said she'd give Jon a decent chance. Why is she trying to spoil our happiness?*

While dinner was cooking, they all sat down in the living room. Karen expected that Jon and her parents would have a relaxing time getting acquainted with each other. But after a few minutes, it was obvious even to Jon that his presence wasn't appreciated by her parents. His face mirrored confusion and hurt feelings. *I should have warned him,* Karen told herself.

Her father even set up rules. "You will not be allowed to stay up after I have gone to bed at night," he said, "and you will not go anywhere by yourselves. Do I make myself clear?"

Jon and Karen nodded their heads, but Karen raged inwardly. She could tell that her parents had planned their strategy well in advance, and she felt thoroughly humiliated. Whatever happened to the terrific people that Jon wanted to meet? How could they treat them this way? Her parents had never been so strict, even when she was engaged to Charles!

After Jon had been in their home for a few days, Karen's father asked to see her in his office, a place reserved only for the most serious discussions. *What's this all about?* she wondered as she entered the room that afternoon.

"Sit down, Karen." His brusque manner puzzled her. Despite the off-and-on friction that she and her mother had had over Jon, Karen felt that her relationship with her father was secure. They had always communicated.

The silence dragged on, and she could tell that her father was having a difficult time beginning the subject on his mind. *It has to be about Jon and me,* Karen guessed, feeling more nervous as the minutes ticked by. But as far as she knew, during the time Jon had been there, they hadn't broken any rules. They hadn't had a chance!

He cleared his throat and finally began to speak. "Karen, do you remember Dave and Cynthia Johnson?"

"Yes, of course." The Johnsons were her parents' old college friends. They visited whenever they came through town on vacations. It was always fun because they had eight children. *But why is he mentioning them?* she wondered.

"Well," his face reddened slightly as he continued, "I don't think you know that Jeff, their oldest son, was conceived before they were married."

I don't like the way this conversation is heading! Karen thought. However, she realized that she didn't have a choice about its direction. Her father was clearly in the driver's seat, so she quickly figured that her best strategy was to say nothing. She'd always admired her father's bluntness—the ability to "get down to brass tacks," as he called it. Now she wasn't so sure about it.

When he failed to get a reaction from her, he went on. "Of course, they didn't mean for it to happen," he explained. "They were in college and planned to marry when Dave graduated. Then Cynthia got pregnant and they quit school to get married. And now, after twenty years of marriage and eight children, Dave has divorced Cynthia and moved in with another woman. Worst of all, he's renounced his faith in Christ."

Karen forgot her intention to keep silent. "But Dad, you can't blame their divorce on the fact that they had to get married," she argued. "How about all those years when they were both Christians? I've heard them share in family devotions, and I know by the way they prayed and acted that they really loved Christ and each other." She shook her head vehemently as she pointed out, "You can't say God is now punishing them twenty years later for a mistake they made in the beginning."

"No, that's true, Karen," he agreed. "What I meant to point out is that there are consequences that follow sin, even though God forgives and forgets. When something like premarital sex happens, there is a loss of trust and respect. Sometimes couples don't completely forgive each other and the relationship never quite heals." He stopped for a moment as if he weren't sure what to say next.

Karen fervently hoped it was the end of that conscience-squirming subject. But her father doggedly kept going. "I just want to warn you that things like this do happen," he said. "It's one of Satan's traps, and sometimes I think he works harder on Christian young people than he does on nonbelievers."

He paused for her comments, but Karen wasn't about to say anything more for fear of incriminating herself. The silence became awkward. She heard the clock ticking loudly. The seconds felt like hours. The air conditioner clicked on, and she felt grateful for its hum. Anything to mask the dreadful quiet!

He sighed deeply and then continued hesitantly, "I don't know if you and Jon have had sexual relations yet. . . ." His voice trailed off into a question mark.

She was thoroughly shocked. How did he guess? Or had he even guessed? She wished she knew. She couldn't answer him. She wouldn't lie—but neither would she admit that he was right.

She tried to look scandalized by his suggestion, but she was afraid that she hadn't succeeded in fooling him. He had always said that her face was an open book, and he was skilled in reading it. Now Karen couldn't look at him, so she studied the titles on his bookshelf.

Finally he spoke, his voice quivering with emotion. "Well, *if* you and Jon have, your mother and I think it would be best for you to get married. You remember that the Apostle Paul said it was better to marry than to burn." He waited for her to acknowledge the biblical quotation. She nodded her head, incapable of speech.

"By the way, I'd like to take a couple of days to go camping with Jon," he said suddenly.

"That would be great! He likes to camp and fish." *Whew!* she thought, relieved to be off such a hot subject.

"I think I need to get to know Jon better, especially since it's possible that he's going to be my son-in-law. He'll probably relax a little if he's out of your mother's company for a while—she needs a rest, too." He grinned then, and she felt that somehow, *maybe,* he understood just a little bit.

"See you later," he dismissed her and she quickly headed for the door. Just as she reached it, he spoke again. "Karen," he added, "I want you to know that we'll always love you, no matter what choices you make. Just remember that, will you?" She thought his eyes looked wet, but perhaps she was mistaken.

"I will, Dad. Thanks, and I love you, too." She retraced her steps and kissed him softly. Then she ran out the door before her inevitable tears began.

I don't think he knows for sure what's going on, she thought. *But what did I do to make him even suspect the truth? The last thing I ever wanted to do was to hurt Mom and Dad—but I'm afraid I already have. The problem is, if they knew what we've done, they'd never* ever *in a million years forgive Jon even if we were married!* She bent her head and cried bitterly. *Nobody understands and there's no one to talk to about this mess!*

For the first time in her life, Karen felt that she couldn't go to her father as her pastor. Her wrong choices had created a wall of distrust between them. She felt that she'd irretrievably lost one of her most precious possessions—clear and honest communication with her parents.

The next morning, her father and Jon left for a two-day camping trip. She missed Jon dreadfully, but was grateful for the decreased tension around the house. However, she and her mother couldn't communicate about much besides housework and her job at the Country Kettle. *If I didn't go to work every day, I don't think I could survive being home,* Karen thought.

She was certain that her parents had talked about the counseling session, and her mother had probably drawn her own conclusions—that Jon was a wolf attacking their dear little Red Riding Hood. *I wonder if Charles wrote them a letter to tip them off.... No,* she decided, *I don't think he'd do something that low.* Though she knew that she and Jon deserved her parents' distrust, she continued to hope that they had somehow fooled them.

Karen wondered how Jon and her father were getting along. Perhaps they'd talk a lot, and maybe her dad would recognize Jon's many good qualities. He'd always been one to give others the benefit of the doubt, even the tramps who came by the church asking for handouts. She giggled when she recalled the X's the hobos had made on the corner of the parsonage to signal others that her father was an easy touch. How many times had he gotten out the paintbrush with Mom standing behind him in frustration? Yet her father continued to believe in people against all odds.

She had little doubt that he would extend that same compassion to Jon. *Everything will be all right,* she reassured herself.

The men returned with stubby beards and a huge string of fish. They seemed to have enjoyed their trip. Now that they were back, however, the battle between her mother and Jon became a full-scale operation.

Perhaps Karen was defensive because of her love for both of them, but it seemed as though her mother picked continually at Jon and that he reacted just as strongly back to her. And the arguments seemed to be over the littlest issues— hardly causes for all-out war.

Karen sighed. Jon's visit had become a miserable nightmare to her. She didn't think she could stand being emotionally pulled apart any longer, and she doubted that her parents were enjoying the situation either.

"Let's go back to Seattle *now*," she suggested to Jon. "Please? We can move into the dorms early. The freshmen are already there for orientation week."

Her parents argued about their early departure plans, but not too strongly. Perhaps they realized the futility of trying to break up her relationship with him.

CHAPTER
6

KAREN smiled and waved good-bye to her parents as she and Jon drove away from the house. When she could no longer see them, she relaxed and settled back for the long drive to Seattle.

"By the way, how did you and Dad get along on the camping trip?" she asked. Due to her parents' close supervision, she and Jon hadn't had much of a chance to discuss anything.

"Everything went fine, except that I got a lecture—a real sizzler!" As he told her the highlights, they discovered that he'd received the identical talk that her father had given to her.

"How did he guess?" Jon wondered aloud, as mystified as she was.

"I don't know. I'm not sure that he did guess. He may have just realized that we're serious about each other, and felt that we should be warned about the dangers involved." She suddenly remembered that Jon had told the retreat speaker all the details of their love life. Surely he hadn't made the same mistake with Dad! "What did you tell him?" she asked nervously.

"I didn't admit anything. In fact, I did a pretty good job of looking dumb, but I'm not sure I fooled him."

Karen stared out the car window as the countryside flashed by. "If he *does* know what we've done," she said slowly, "I doubt that you fooled him, either. I'm afraid that I didn't carry the act too well myself. But what are we going to do now? Should we go ahead and get married?" Paul's famous line, "It's better to marry than to burn," echoed in her mind. But no matter what her father had said, she still didn't feel that her parents wanted them to marry yet—"don't burn" was more like it.

Jon, his eyes still on the road, managed to give her a quick kiss. "Sure," he agreed readily. "Are you ready to announce our engagement?"

"Yes, but *when* do you think we can get married?"

"I think we should wait at least until I graduate in June," he replied. "It takes a lot of money to get married, and I've seen too many guys quit with one quarter to go. They're forever trying to make it up so they can graduate."

"I suppose you're right." She sighed with disappointment. "I was hoping we could have the wedding during Christmas break, but I guess it just wouldn't work."

"What's the rush? We've planned all along to wait until after graduation."

Karen picked nervously at the upholstery. "I'm

just afraid that we'll get into trouble," she finally admitted. "Then what?"

Jon didn't say anything for a minute. He frowned as he thought it over. "We've made it for three months," he pointed out.

"Sure! By being away from each other! That doesn't mean anything." A note of sarcasm had crept into her voice.

"Yes, but it does prove we can live without it. We don't *need* to have sex until we're married. All it takes is willpower," he insisted. "We'll just spend our time in other ways—like studying, for one!"

"I'd feel a whole lot better if we did get more involved in school," she agreed. "After all, that's why we're there."

Once they arrived on campus, they settled into their new quarters. To Karen's delight, she and Tricia were roommates again.

"Wow! Is this ever a step up from Flanders Hall!" she exclaimed as she dumped her suitcases in the doorway to their room. The earth-toned plush carpeting and crisp white walls provided an easy color scheme to work with, and they soon decorated it to their taste.

Jon moved into a college-owned apartment with his friends Brad and Mike. He found a new job in a warehouse that paid good wages. Even so, he barely made enough to pay for the increased tuition costs and other expenses. "I could starve to death," he joked, "especially with Brad's cooking!"

Karen went back to work at her old part-time job as a waitress. "Same old thing," she complained to Tricia. "At least you got a new job—an easy one, too! You just check to make sure that all the little chickadees are tucked into bed. You're a glorified mother hen!" she teased.

"It's not that simple," Tricia replied, defending her job. "I have to worry over all the late ones, and if they're late three times, I have to report them and they can be suspended. I won't have any friends left," she moaned.

"I'll still love you, Trish. And I promise not to give you wrinkles and gray hair!"

"I wouldn't worry about you anyway," Tricia commented with a smile. "And I won't report you if you're late. You and Jon would never do anything you aren't supposed to. If you can't trust a preacher's kid and a student minister, who can you trust?"

For a while Karen and Jon were so busy that Tricia's faith in them was justified. Between their jobs, classes, school activities, and his basketball practices, their time seemed completely filled. The band began rehearsing for concerts and parades, too.

"I can hardly keep up," Karen told Jon over a stack of reference books in the library. It was mid-December and they were working on term papers. Both of them were doing better in their classes, but Karen often looked exhausted and pale. "All we ever do is study and work," she said wearily.

"You're right," Jon agreed. "We haven't even had time for a date in weeks. It's been a real grind." He pushed back his chair and stood up.

"Let's go out to dinner," he suggested. "We deserve a break."

"That sounds super!" Karen smiled gratefully and went to dress for the occasion.

Later that evening as they were finishing their desserts, she noticed again just how handsome Jon was, especially in the romantic candlelight. She glowed as she thought of all his endearing qualities.

"What do you want to do now, Karen?" he asked. "We have a while until curfew."

"Wel-l-l," she drawled, "if I had my druthers, I'd want to kiss you!" She winked at him and giggled.

"You want to go park?"

"Don't be gross! I said I want to *kiss* you. Can't we trust each other that much?"

"I guess in the last six months we've proven that we can behave ourselves. Are you ready to leave?" He stood up and held Karen's chair for her, then carefully assisted her with her coat.

They headed for their favorite park, always deserted during winter evenings. The wind blew ferociously and the rain beat against the windshield, but they were toasty warm inside the car, thanks to the heater. They talked about their marriage plans, stopping to kiss once in a while.

Then Jon turned the key, shutting off the heater and windshield wipers. "We're going to run out of gas if I keep all this going," he explained.

Karen didn't mind, and snuggled into his arms. *We'll be careful,* she promised herself.

77

Jon kissed her tenderly at first, but each kiss became more insistent, more passionate. She responded eagerly as long-buried impulses rose within her. *We're going too far—too far,* she warned herself.

All too soon they were locked in their old trap, controlled by their sexual desires. *Stop!* Karen's mind screamed. And then suddenly she didn't care anymore, as she surrendered to her passions.

But when it was over, she was ashamed and angry—mostly with herself. *That was so stupid!* she thought. *Now look what we've done and it was all my idea. I was the one who suggested coming up here!* She glanced up at Jon and saw that his face looked grim.

"I'm sorry, Karen." He sighed heavily and tears came into his eyes. "I was so sure that we could handle it—but I should have known better. I never should have brought you up here."

"It's all right. What happened was my fault."

"No, it's *my* fault. I'm responsible for what happens to you, and I really blew it." His hands clenched the steering wheel. "I hate myself," he said bitterly.

"Don't, Jon. Don't say that! I love you and I know how you feel. I feel the same way—rotten."

"I love you, too, Karen, and I know that I've hurt you. It isn't worth that."

She was dismayed as she saw that he was crying. And then she couldn't control her tears either as she hugged him close to her.

"What time is it?" he asked suddenly. He

turned on the dome light and glanced at his watch. "We're late!" he groaned as he started the car.

Karen didn't answer. It didn't matter, she thought. Tricia wouldn't report her. . . .

December passed quickly as Karen studied for finals and tried to keep up with the hectic holiday activities. She went home to visit her parents during Christmas, while Jon flew to New Jersey to be with his father.

Two weeks later they were back at college to begin the next term. Though Karen didn't feel well most of the time, she tried to ignore it. But the dizziness and nausea just wouldn't go away. *I'm almost sure it's not the flu*, she worried. *I think I'm pregnant. . . . Or maybe it's just my imagination again.* She tried to push her suspicions to the back of her mind.

Jon found her daydreaming in the music building one afternoon. She was supposed to be practicing the clarinet. "Come on," he said. "Let's go get something to eat. Mike's cooking tonight, and I can't stand to eat it—whatever it is!"

"OK," she agreed readily and put her instrument away.

They chose a nearby family restaurant. "Order anything you want, Karen," Jon said as they looked at the menu. "I'm rich this week—especially since I have *you*." He leaned over to kiss her. "You're the best thing that ever happened to me."

Karen smiled weakly. *I wonder if he'll still think that when he finds out . . .* , she worried. She read through the selections again, trying to find something that she thought might taste good. "I'm not very hungry," she said finally. "Do you mind if I just have a dinner salad?"

"What's the matter? You aren't sick, are you?"

"No . . . I don't think so. I'm just not hungry, and there's no point in wasting your money. But I'm enjoying being here with you, so go ahead and order big."

"Are you sure you're not sick?" he asked.

She shook her head and panicked as waves of nausea rolled in her stomach. She pushed back her chair and stood up. "Be back in a minute," she mumbled as she fled to the restroom.

How long can I keep this a secret? she thought as she vomited. *Jon's sure to guess, and Tricia won't be far behind. What am I going to do?* She tried to regain her composure before going out to face him again.

"You OK?" he asked. "You were sure gone a long time."

She didn't answer, and poked at her salad as she felt suddenly on the verge of tears.

If Jon noticed her discomfiture, he didn't acknowledge it as he silently finished his dinner. "Ready to go?" he asked abruptly. "I'll take you home."

He's angry, Karen thought. *And it's because I've ruined our evening.* Tears squeezed out from behind her tightly closed eyelids. *I suppose I may as well finish it off, since we're both miserable already.*

"I'm not ready to go home," she told him as they walked out the restaurant door. "I need to talk about something."

"That's fine with me. You haven't talked all evening," he replied sarcastically.

They got into the car, and he looked searchingly at her. "I'm sorry," he apologized. "It's just that I know something is bothering you, and you won't tell me what it is. All the guessing I've been doing has really bugged me. Have I said or done something to upset you?"

"No. . . ." She glanced up at him and then away. *What if he won't love me anymore?* she thought anxiously. "I hate to tell you this," she began, "but I—I'm pregnant." She stopped. It sounded so cold, so blunt . . . so final.

Jon's face blanched. "What? Are you sure? Have you seen a doctor? Why didn't you tell me before now?"

"Yes, I'm sure. No, I haven't seen a doctor. And I was afraid to tell you—that's why I haven't said anything."

"But you thought you were pregnant last time," he pointed out. "And you weren't."

"I am this time," she insisted stubbornly. "I can tell. Don't ask me how I know—I just do." Her hands were balled up into tight little fists in her lap. "And I don't need any doctor," she added fiercely.

"You have to see a doctor, Karen. If you want, I'll take you to someone besides Dr. Miller."

"No, I won't go!" she cried, and then all the pent-up worry and terror broke loose as she wept on his shoulder. "What am I going to do? I can't have a baby! We'll get kicked out of school and my parents will never forgive us—oh, Jon. . . ."

"Hush, Karen. It'll all work out." He held her as he tried awkwardly to comfort her. "Honey, no matter what happens, I'll always love you," he reassured her. "Nothing can ever change that." He kissed her tenderly. "You belong to me, and I belong to you. If you're going to have a baby— so am I. We're in this together, OK?"

"OK, but if we're in this together, then what are *we* going to do? I don't know *what* to do, Jon!"

"Don't get excited—I'll think of something. I just need some time to get used to the idea." He silently considered the dilemma. "Let's just get married now," he suggested finally. "We'll just move the date up a few months."

"A few months!" Karen exclaimed. "We may as well advertise on the front page that we have to get married! My dad would resign and probably leave the ministry. Besides that, the church would never let you be a pastor—and that's what God called you to do. You've just spent the last four years preparing for it!"

Jon nodded. "You're right," he agreed. "And things wouldn't be so great with my folks, either. Mom would eventually adjust, but Dad would disown me—he said he would."

He slumped down over the steering wheel. "Besides that," he added, "we'd be expelled from school, and even though we could enroll somewhere else, it probably would be next to impossible to get scholarships. To top it off, I'm supposed to graduate in a few months—this will wreck everything!"

"There's no sense in both of us messing up

our lives," she thought out loud. "If I left and went someplace. . . ."

"Don't you dare even think about taking off!" he exploded. "I said we're in this together, and I mean it! I love you, Karen, and I'm not about to lose you no matter what the consequences are. It's my fault, too, and I deserve whatever comes. If I could, I'd take all the heat. I hate the thought of you suffering through any of this."

He kissed her forehead. "But stop your worrying, honey. There has to be an answer somewhere."

"We'd better get home. It's getting late," she replied in a tired, hollow voice.

The next afternoon, Jon caught up with her as she headed for her sociology class. "Come on, Karen," he said. "I made a doctor's appointment for you at three o'clock."

"I'm not going! I told you I didn't want to see a doctor!"

"You're going—and that's all there is to it."

Karen sighed. She was too tired to argue with him and she supposed he was right. "It's not Dr. Miller?" She certainly wasn't going back *there*— not after he'd warned them.

"No, I called a doctor in downtown Seattle. Is that far enough away from the college to suit you?"

"All right, let's get it over with," she agreed unwillingly.

An hour later, they sat fidgeting in the waiting room. Karen noted the ripped vinyl upholstery and the spots on the carpet. Most of the magazines were coverless and dog-eared, and the plants were either drooping or dead. Her opinion of the doctor declined each minute they waited.

"How did you ever pick a dump like this?" she asked Jon.

"I couldn't tell from the phone book listing." His tone was acid. But then his face softened as he noticed her distressed look. "Hey, I don't like it anymore than you do, but it'll be over soon. Everything will be OK—don't worry," he tried to reassure her.

The nurse stood at the door. "Karen Blackburn," she called.

Karen blushed. Did she have to say it so loud? She resisted the impulse to ignore the summons, and followed the nurse to the tiny cubicle.

The doctor strode in almost as soon as Karen was seated. "Well, what are you here for?" he asked brusquely.

"I—I think I'm pregnant," she faltered, choking on the unpleasant words.

The doctor gave her a bored, "I've-seen-this-a-million-times-before" look. "I'll send the nurse in with a specimen container," he said. "You can call the office in three days." He turned on his heel and left, closing the door sharply behind him.

Terrific bedside manner, Karen thought bitterly, but then supposed that she deserved it. After all, she couldn't expect him to turn cartwheels for another pregnant teenager....

Three days later she called the doctor's office from a telephone booth. "Karen Blackburn?" the voice answered. "Just a minute, I'll check....

Miss Blackburn? Yes, you are pregnant. Good-bye." Karen heard the click on the other end of the line, and hung up the receiver wordlessly. She walked over to the car where Jon waited.

"It's official," she said flatly as she climbed in. She leaned back against the seat and closed her eyes. She was almost too tired to face the situation or to care that she was in it. Everything seemed entirely beyond her control.

Jon, however, was trying to come to grips with the problem. "What are we going to do now?" he demanded. "You don't want to get married—so what's left?"

"I *do* want to get married, but not this way. It would ruin your chances of ever being a minister, and then there are our families to consider, and—we've been over this ground before. Besides that, I don't ever want you to feel like you *have* to marry me. It takes all the joy out of it." She wept bitterly.

"I *want* to marry you," he emphasized, "and I'd never feel roped into it. We chose each other a long time ago. Nothing will change that. But you're right," he agreed. "Getting married this way would blow everything and cause a lot of grief." He held her eyes with a determined gaze. "But there's one thing we have to face, Karen. Either you are going to have a baby or you're not going to have it."

"I hardly have a choice, do I?" She wiped her tears as she thought about it. "That is, unless I would have a miscarriage. . . . Do you think we could pray for one? I know it sounds awful, but I don't think it's exactly God's will for us to have this baby, and it would solve the problem. . . ."

Jon looked doubtful. "I don't think God is going to cause a miscarriage for our convenience. We can take the consequences and either get married or give the baby up for adoption." He leaned forward and nervously drummed his fingers on the dashboard as he watched the cars whiz by.

"Adoption! You must be kidding! There's no way I'd give up my baby to someone else. It would be yours and mine—part of us! I couldn't do that—I just couldn't." She felt alone in her terror and confusion. Not even Jon had any answers this time, she thought in despair.

"Karen. . . ." His tone was tentative, hesitant. "There is another way. . . ."

Hope kindled in her eyes. "What are you talking about?" she asked impatiently.

But he remained silent, staring down at the brake pedal as though it held the illusive answer to their problem. Finally he quietly suggested, "You could get an abortion. . . ."

Karen recoiled as if he'd physically struck her. "Jon! How could you even say that?" she cried. "It's completely out of the question. You don't care about me at all!"

"I do *too* care about you," he insisted. "But I was talking with a guy down at the plant, and he said that his girl friend had just had one and that Welfare had paid for it."

"But why would Welfare pay for it, and what good would it do me, anyway? I'm not on Welfare!"

"You don't have to already be on Welfare to

get one free," he patiently explained. "You just have to show them that you can't afford to pay for one, and then they'll pick up the bill."

"I don't know, Jon. I don't really understand abortion. I don't know what my parents would think about it—I don't even know what *I* think."

He shrugged. "Well, you know what they would think about your being pregnant. . : ."

Karen still felt unconvinced. *But maybe we should look into it,* she reasoned. "How do we find out about this—this abortion?" she asked, wishing there were a substitute for the ugly word.

"He said that they called a family planning agency. They're supposed to know how to take care of this kind of problem. Do you want to check it out?"

Karen wasn't sure. She'd had a hard enough time just accepting the fact that she was pregnant. Now she had to try to cope with the idea that she could change that fact legally and safely—if she wanted to. "Well, maybe," she said at last, her tone doubtful. "It looks as if it might be our only alternative to get out of this mess. And if no one finds out what we've done, it *will* avoid a lot of heartache."

"Even so, I think we should think about this overnight. It's a big decision to make," Jon pointed out.

"Overnight? Don't we have more time than that?" She suddenly felt as though she were about to suffocate from the weight of the deci- sion. "I don't know, Jon . . . I just don't know. Wouldn't we be doing something really wrong? I mean, aren't we talking about our baby?" She looked him straight in the eye.

He nodded. "I guess there aren't any right answers to sin," he admitted. "Maybe we should get some counseling. Do you want to talk to someone at the church? Maybe Larry and Janie?" he suggested suddenly.

She shook her head. "I don't want *anyone* to know if I can help it," she said.

Jon shrugged. "OK," he agreed. "It won't be an easy thing to decide, and I don't want to pressure you. The guy did say, though, that it should be done within the first three months of pregnancy or it becomes a lot more complicated. We don't have much time left."

He sighed deeply as he started the car. "We'd better get back to the college. I have a lot of studying to do tonight—if I can concentrate on it."

They pulled up in front of her dormitory a few minutes later, and he kissed her goodnight. "Try not to worry too much tonight," he told her. "It won't do any good, and you need to get some rest. I'll see you in the morning."

She ran to her room and closed the door behind her as hot tears spilled down her cheeks. Thank goodness Tricia was gone, she thought, holding her aching head in her hands. She kicked off her shoes and curled up on her bed, but sleep eluded her. Instead, she spent the night nibbling soda crackers and trying to fight down the nausea that continually rose in her throat. Her secret twisted inside her as she grappled with the decision of what to do next.

Jon's right, she finally concluded. *There are no right answers. Whatever we decide is going to be wrong and it will hurt somebody—the questions are "who?" and "how badly?"* The weight of that knowledge crushed her spirit. *I can't choose! I just can't!* And then she sobbed brokenly, "I wish I were dead. . . ."

CHAPTER
7

"I'VE thought it over," Karen told Jon after their first class the next morning. "I want to call the family planning agency, but I don't want to use any of the phones around here."

"Let's go find a phone booth then," he suggested.

They drove down several streets before he spotted one and pulled over. "Here's some change," he said, handing it to her.

"I've got to hurry or I'll be late for work," she said as she jumped out of the car. She closeted herself inside the booth and flipped nervously through the Yellow Pages. She called the first family planning agency on the list, hoping she'd chosen the right one.

Karen tearfully tried to explain her problem to the woman who answered the phone. She seemed to be understanding, and Karen immediately felt that the woman was on her side. *This is going to work out,* she told herself, feeling greatly relieved. *I'm finally going to get an answer to this mess.*

Just then the woman asked, "Do you have any money? It costs five hundred dollars."

Karen's stomach lurched and nausea overcame her. Where would they get the money? It might as well have been a million dollars—she didn't have anything but what she'd saved for next term's tuition, and neither did Jon. She thought he'd said that Welfare would pay for it!

"How about your parents?" the receptionist suggested.

"But I *can't* tell them! They would never pay for an abortion." She began to cry, terrified that the agency might contact her family.

"Well, you are legally on your own since your parents are paying less than half your support, and you do not live in their home. I'll give you the telephone number of the district attorney. You just tell him what you've told me. I'm sure everything will work out fine," she said reassuringly.

Karen thanked her and hung up the phone. Then she dialed the district attorney's number and once again explained her story. He, too, was kind, friendly, and supportive.

"Are you and your young man planning to get married later?" he asked, and seemed pleased when she answered yes.

"Just stick together through this," he counseled, and then told her that he would authorize the state to pay for the abortion. "You'll have to go down to the Welfare office to fill out the necessary forms, however."

Relieved at how smoothly everything seemed to be fitting together, she thanked him and hung up the phone. Just then, a sharp knock on the door of the phone booth startled her, and she wheeled around to face Mike. *Why did Jon have to pick a spot right next to the store where Mike works?* she angrily blamed Jon as she suddenly recognized the location. She hoped she looked nonchalant as she pushed open the door.

"What are you doing calling from a phone booth, Karen?" he asked. "Why waste a quarter when you can call from the dorm—or isn't it private enough for you?"

Dismayed, she wondered how long Mike had been standing there. Had he heard anything? Guiltily she retorted, "Mind your own business!"

"Hey, I was just teasing you!" He looked quizzically at her. "You seem worried, Karen. Anything I can do to help?"

She shook her head, fighting back tears as Mike walked with her toward the car where Jon was waiting. *Jon looks so nervous,* she thought, and then added bitterly, *well, he ought to! Why didn't he sidetrack Mike instead of letting him stand over there eavesdropping on me! What a dummy!*

"What's going on?" Mike asked Jon point-blank.

Jon and Karen looked helplessly at each other, and then Jon shrugged his shoulders. "Want to tell him, Karen?" he asked.

Her heart pounded furiously as she thought,

Now you've done it, Jon Hamilton! But Mike *was* a good listener, she knew, from what Jon had told her. They were prayer partners and often shared confidences. *Oh, well. Now that he knows something's wrong, he'll get it out of us sooner or later,* she reasoned.

She suddenly felt unable to hold the turmoil inside any longer, and she began to sob through their miserable story, hoping that Mike would understand their problem and the decision they'd had to make. "I've decided to have an abortion," she told him, noting the half-surprised look on Jon's face. Karen in turn was surprised. *He didn't think I'd really do it,* she realized.

"You're crazy!" Mike shouted. "You can't kill a baby!"

Karen was shocked. She hadn't expected the angry venom in Mike's voice. "B-b-but we *aren't* killing a baby, Mike. That's one of the questions I asked the family planning agency—"

"Family planning agency—ha!" Mike spat out the words. "Family *killing* agency is more like it!"

"Mike—" Jon's tone had a warning edge to it. "Just pipe down and listen. This isn't easy for us, you know."

"Sure it's easy for you! You aren't kidding me!" Mike's voice dripped sarcasm.

"Mike," Karen tried again. "Let me finish. I talked to several people today, and each one said that it was the best plan for us. We aren't ready to get married. Jon still has to graduate and we don't have any money, and we have to consider our families and—"

"Have you considered your families?" Mike interrupted. "*Really* considered them? Do you honestly know how they'd feel about this?"

She tried to explain to Mike about their parents' viewpoints and the harm that would come if they knew about her pregnancy. "Besides, Mike, these people said that we're only getting rid of an unwanted, unplanned mass of cells. It's really just contraception after the fact instead of before," she assured him, still hoping that she could make him understand.

"I don't buy that," he stated vehemently. "I think you should talk to your parents. In fact, I don't understand how you got yourselves into this mess in the first place." He stood silently beside the car for a moment, his face tight with anger and shock as he sorted through his thoughts. Finally he said contemptuously, "All I can say is, you're both phonies. God will never use you— for anything!" Then he slammed the car door and strode away.

They watched him disappear into the store. Then Jon turned to her and breathed a long, deep, hopeless sigh—almost a groan. "I thought Mike would understand," he said, "but I know now that we can never talk to *anyone* about this."

Karen knew that he was hurt far more than she was by Mike's statements. Mike was his special, close friend. *It's all my fault—I should have kept my mouth shut*, she told herself. *Jon's right, though. If we can't trust Mike, then we can't trust any of our friends or family to understand.*

"Shall we go through with it?" she asked him, afraid that after what Mike said, he might have changed his mind.

"What did the agency have to say?" he asked. She outlined the calls she'd made and the steps they had to take.

"Let's go then," Jon decided. "No sense dragging this out. I'll take you to the Welfare office right now. You'd better call work and tell them you'll be a little late."

Karen felt grateful that he'd offered to go with her to the Welfare office. She certainly didn't want to face that hurdle by herself. But nothing, not even Jon by her side, could prepare her for the psychological shock of that place. It was more than an office—it was an environment, totally foreign to her and far worse than she'd ever imagined.

Her shocked eyes took in the green painted concrete block walls and the ugly posters advising them of criminal penalties for misuse of food stamps and Welfare funds. Tired women with scarred, bare legs, and bleary-eyed drunks waited in an endless zigzag line that led to the information desk.

Karen joined the line, feeling conspicuous as angry eyes seemed to probe and question, "What are *you* doing here?" She realized uncomfortably that she was better dressed than most of the people. Little children, a few barefoot even in the cold January weather, cried and fought.

"Can't we go home, Mommy?" a little boy sobbed. "I'm hungry."

"Shut up!" the woman hissed. "There's nothin' to eat there, anyway."

Karen began to cry. She cried for the little boy and his mother. She cried for the barefoot children. She cried for her own shame and despair. She felt still worse for penalizing the hard-working taxpayers.

After giving her name and the nature of her business to the receptionist, she found Jon and sat beside him on an orange plastic seat as she waited her turn. She winced as the loudspeaker blared, "Karen Blackburn."

Why didn't I give them a phony name? she thought, suddenly terrified. *Now it'll be on my record—anyone might pry. What if the government wants an abortion survey ten years from now and decides to track me down?* She shuddered at the thought as she went to meet the woman who was waiting for her.

"Hello, Karen," the caseworker greeted her with a smile. "Let's use this office." She pointed to a desk and two chairs, separated from other similar areas with only bulletin board partitions.

Not much privacy, Karen thought as she clearly heard other interviews taking place.

"You'll need to fill out this application first, and then I'll be back to ask some questions," the woman told her. She left as Karen stared at the pages of information she was required to give the state.

Most of it was financial data, she realized. "List your assets. Do you have more than five hundred dollars? Do you own a car worth more than one thousand dollars? What is your salary? Do you have a savings account? Are you a home-owner or a renter? Do you receive income other than a salary?"

Wow! Karen thought. *Where does college fit into all this? Do I count my scholarship money? How much do I put down for rent and utilities? Where does my tuition expense go on this budget?*

Karen found out the hard answers to those questions when the caseworker returned. "I'm sorry," she said, "but your college expenses do not qualify as valid budget items. In fact, you will have to either quit school or your job to get an abortion if you expect the state to pay for it."

"What? But I don't understand!"

"You have two choices, Karen. You can quit school and use the money you earn from your job to pay for your abortion—since you don't have enough to pay for both. Or you can quit your job so that you will financially qualify for aid to pay for the abortion," she explained. "Either way, it looks as though you lose out on college—at least for a while. I'm sorry, but that's the rule."

Then she glanced again at the application. "Oh, I see that you didn't finish. I'll need this in-formation. What is your mother's maiden name? Who is your father? When and where was he born?" She scribbled in Karen's answers, gaining a complete family history.

Does she really have to know all that? Karen wondered, afraid that Welfare would contact her parents to make them pay for the abortion or to give permission.

"Can your family supply the money for the abortion?" the caseworker asked.

"No," Karen answered quickly and then explained that she didn't intend for her parents to find out about the abortion. "You won't tell them, will you?" she asked anxiously.

"No, of course not. This is all confidential information."

As the interview continued, Karen was surprised that neither Jon nor his family were considered as potential money sources by Welfare. Not that they were an actual solution, but it was the principle of the thing.

Finally, the caseworker pressed Karen for a decision. "You'll have to either quit school to pay the abortion costs yourself, or quit your job so that we can assume responsibility. There is no other way, Karen."

"I understand, but I'll have to talk to Jon first," Karen replied. She was dangerously close to tears.

"Fine, but call me as soon as you can. The sooner the abortion is done, the safer it is for the mother," she said as she ushered Karen from her office.

Mother. The term pierced her conscience. *Am I really a mother?* Karen certainly didn't feel like one. She told herself that she had no child, only an egg, still unformed, like any of a thousand inside her body. It was a mistake, nothing more.

Convincing herself for the moment, she felt better... except for the money problem. How was she going to pay for the abortion?

"What'll we do now?" She put the question to Jon a few minutes later as they sat in the car discussing the situation.

"Karen, it's really up to you. But if you want my opinion, I think you should quit your job. You can get another one after the abortion—say, in a few weeks."

"But how will I make up my lost wages? And what if I can't find another job?"

"We'll cross that when we get there—maybe with another loan or something," he suggested.

Karen nodded. "I guess you're right. I'll go tell the caseworker what we've decided. Wait here!" She hurried back into the building.

A few minutes passed, and then she came back out and got into the car. "Jon, can you take me to another appointment?" she asked. "Don't worry about my job—I just called and they fired me for being late." She shrugged. "I guess it saved me the trouble of quitting."

"When's the appointment? I don't want to lose *my* job. Then we'll really be in a fix!"

"It's at one o'clock."

"Sure, I'll take you. I don't go to work until six tonight. That should leave enough time." She gave him directions, and they headed for the last interview.

At one o'clock sharp, Karen stood uncertainly in the doorway of the county hospital administrator's office. His steely eyes bored into hers, and she nervously averted her glance, at the same time instinctively reaching for Jon's hand to steady herself. "Oh, God, I'm so scared," she prayed, feeling desperate, but yet doubting that he heard her or cared. *Not now,* she thought miserably. *I've gone too far away to ask for his help.* She stood frozen in her thoughts until Jon nudged her.

"Sit down." The man's brusque tone was an order, not an invitation. They quickly obeyed, hoping that the session would be short and painless. But instead, he ignored their presence and seemed to be examining some papers in a folder on his desk.

The silence stretched before them like the timeline to eternity. Karen felt confused and uneasy. She studied the plush carpeting, glanced at the memorabilia on his desk, and debated whether or not the plants were real. *Am I supposed to talk first?* she wondered, and chanced a quick look at the administrator. She was shocked at his angry countenance. Her stomach twisted and churned.

"You really have a lot of nerve," he finally spat out disgustedly. Tears flooded Karen's eyes, and she bit her lip, trying desperately to keep her emotions under control. *This is worse than I ever dreamed,* she told herself. But then she suddenly realized that he was addressing Jon—not her. For he was saying, "How could you come into this office, under these conditions, wearing your school jacket? If I were you, at least I'd have the decency not to smear my school's name, too."

Jon choked on some words and then gave up.

He'd forgotten, Karen supposed, or perhaps never realized the implications of wearing their school's insignia. Karen felt as ashamed and guilty as Jon looked. He squirmed as the man silently waited. Visibly shaken, Jon finally removed his jacket.

The administrator continued then, asking all the same questions that the previous interviewers had covered. Karen knew the routine so well by that time that she could answer mechanically and unemotionally.

"My job," he told her, "is to determine whether there is a valid reason under state law why you should have an abortion. The only reason I can possibly give is that motherhood will psychologically harm you at this point in your life. However, I cannot tell how much the *abortion* will harm you now and in the future. I will give permission, but—" he sighed and shook his head before continuing, "I hope you will think over your decision very carefully."

He reluctantly signed the form and handed it to Karen. "Take this up to the third floor," he said as he dismissed them. "They'll begin the process. Then be here tomorrow morning at six."

As the elevator whisked Jon and Karen to the third floor, she wondered what lay ahead. What did the administrator mean by "begin the process"? The elevator door opened to a waiting room jammed with pregnant women. The scene unnerved Jon, who decided to wait downstairs in the main lobby.

Karen handed the form to the receptionist

who glanced briefly at it. "Go to room sixty-seven down the hall," she said. "Some women are already there waiting. A nurse will be in shortly to explain the process and to answer your questions."

Karen found the room and chose a seat. The women sat silently, each alone with her thoughts. The irony of the close-mouthed women struck Karen. They all had one thing in common, she mused, but no one would ever open up to discuss it. *I wonder if any of them are as scared as I am.* She searched their faces for clues, but found none.

Then a young nurse entered, and the women became instantly alert. Just like a roomful of students when the professor arrives, Karen observed in momentary amusement. All that was missing was the sound of textbooks opening and notebooks being readied to record pertinent facts.

The nurse outlined the procedure. "You will each have a gynecological examination immediately following this orientation," she began.

Karen's mind began to float away at the word "orientation." She remembered her freshman initiation week at Wellington. *Why, these women and I are in the process of becoming a select club, a sorority, because of our common experience,* she thought, easily making the symbolic transfer from academics to abortion.

The air seemed stifling to Karen as the nurse droned on. "I want you to understand that an abortion is a major surgical operation," she pointed out. "There is a risk of death. You will be required to sign papers stating that you understand this, and that the hospital will not be held liable in this event."

Death? Karen hadn't considered that possibility. *What if I die?* she thought, quickly panicking. *It's not worth that, and it would be a terrible shock to Mom and Dad.* She almost got up and ran from the room. But the nurse allayed her fear by saying that more women die in childbirth than in legal abortions. Death was a remote possibility.

The nurse went on to explain that as a part of the examination, each woman's uterus would be packed with sterile cotton. This would trigger the opening of the cervix to prepare for the abortion of the fetus the next morning. "You will feel contractions," she said, "much like those when a women is in labor."

Uterus, cervix, contractions, labor? Karen wondered what the terms meant. She didn't remember much of that fourth grade lecture from her mother, and she hadn't troubled herself to find out much since then. The parts of her body and their functions were still mysterious and confusing to her. But she noticed that no one else asked any questions. *I must be the only ignorant one here,* she assumed.

As she tried to digest the medical terms and information, she began to think again about dying. *Maybe I'll be the minor statistic,* she worried. *After all, if God wants to punish me, he has plenty of good reasons.* First, she decided, he could punish her for having had sex with Jon before marriage. She had known all

along what the Bible says—that it's fornication—
and nothing could ever make that right, no matter how much they loved each other. Then, too,
he might punish her for having an abortion, she
guessed. But then she didn't really have a choice
in the matter. Besides, she reassured herself, it's
not a baby yet. She envisioned the shapeless
mass of cells that had been described to her by
the woman from the family planning agency.

I'm glad I'm having the abortion so early,
she told herself. It would be different if she were
five or six months pregnant—then there would
be a child inside her, not just the egg that was
there now.

"In conclusion," the nurse said, "we want to
make sure that none of you will repeat your mistake. The state allows only two abortions, and
many of you have already had one."

You won't have to worry about me! Karen
told her silently.

"We feel that education is the answer," the
nurse continued. "I'm going to explain all the
available contraceptives to you, and you will be
asked to choose one. After your abortion tomorrow, the hospital will send your choice home
with you. It is free, and you are eligible for future supplies if you have financial need. Abortion
must not be viewed as a means of contraception." She looked at each of the women in turn
to make sure her point had penetrated.

What a course in sex education, Karen
thought, wishing it had been available long before then. *Maybe I would have made better
choices.* But she had to admit that Dr. Larson

and Dr. Miller had both tried to educate her. She hadn't given them much of a chance, though, because she was too embarrassed to discuss the subject. And besides, she and Jon were already in far too deep by the time the doctors had come on the scene.

Karen had been right about one thing, she realized. What she didn't know *had* indeed hurt her. How deep the wounds would eventually become, she couldn't know or even guess.

But I won't use the contraceptive, she vowed. *I don't care if I never have sex again after what I've gone through.*

After the painful and humiliating gynecological examination, Karen headed for the elevator. *The sooner I get out of here the better,* she told herself. She quickly found Jon downstairs in the lobby. As they walked toward the exit, she felt physically and emotionally exhausted.

Safe at last in the car, she began to sob, overwhelmed by the day's events. Jon kissed her tenderly. "Just go ahead and cry, honey," he said. "It'll make you feel better to get it out of your system." He started the motor. "We'd better go, though. I have to be at work by six."

Mrs. Thompson, the resident dorm mother, was waiting when Karen walked into the building. "Hello, Karen," she said. "Tricia mentioned to me that you weren't feeling well last night. How are you doing today?"

"Fine," Karen lied.

"You look a little peaked. Have you had dinner?"

Karen shook her head. She was hungry now

that Mrs. Thompson mentioned it, but the cafeteria was closed.

"How about some chicken noodle soup? It usually tastes good if you're feeling under the weather. Why don't you come over to my apartment for a while? I'd like some company."

Karen accepted with reservations. After all, she barely knew Mrs. Thompson. But she hadn't eaten since breakfast, and her mouth watered for some of that soup.

As Karen ate, Mrs. Thompson sipped a cup of tea. "I feel like watching TV," she said. "Would you like to watch it, too?" Karen nodded politely.

Mrs. Thompson frowned as she consulted the guide. "Oh, dear, they've canceled my favorite show. I guess we'll watch the special instead." She switched on the television and then settled herself in the big recliner as the title flashed on the screen.

Oh no! Surely she won't watch this! Karen thought as she realized that the topic was abortion. She wanted to leave, but felt a little awkward about the situation. For openers, she still had a full bowl of soup.

For some unaccountable reason, Mrs. Thompson was interested in the program, and quickly became indignant as her Christian views seemed under attack.

"Karen, can you imagine that?" she sputtered. "How could any woman kill her baby? I would have given everything I owned to be able to have a child."

An awful thought struck Karen forcibly: What

if God would decide to punish her by never allowing her to have a child?

Then Mrs. Jones interrupted her thoughts with more painful questions. "What kind of a woman would do such a thing?" Mrs. Jones clearly felt that either the woman was mentally unbalanced or immoral.

"But what if the woman isn't married?" Karen responded weakly. "What if she has been raped, or having a baby would injure her health?" She tried to think of all the reasons that would justify abortion. There were a few more to go. "Suppose she doesn't want the child or can't financially care for it?"

"Well, yes. . . ." Mrs. Thompson seemed dubious. "But if a woman behaves like that, she should have to bear the child anyway and then give it up for adoption. Someone *else* would gladly love the baby and care for it." She delivered her final round of ammunition, "That doesn't excuse murder!"

Murder. Could I really be guilty of murdering a child? No, she told herself again. *It's only a shapeless blob—that's what the pamphlet said. This is no more murder than using a contraceptive. The only difference is that I'm preventing a pregnancy after instead of before it occurred,* she reminded herself.

But does that difference matter? she wondered as she tossed in her bed that night, unable to sleep. The contractions came in hard, excruciatingly painful waves. *Will morning ever come?* she wondered despairingly. She wrestled again with the perpetual question about abortion.

108

Is it really only a last-minute method of contraception? She desperately wanted to believe that it was. But soon the ordeal would be over, and Karen told herself that she would no longer have to debate whether it was right or wrong. *What a relief that will be,* she thought as the pale gray hint of dawn peeked over the horizon.

CHAPTER

8

"ARE you sure you want to go through with this?" Jon asked Karen as they walked to the parking lot. "It's not too late to change your mind."

She shivered in the cold, foggy morning air. "Yes," she answered firmly, "we've already decided, Jon, and I won't back out now." She thought she detected a measure of relief on his face. *He actually was afraid that I'd change my mind at the last minute!* she realized.

Thoroughly chilled by the time they reached the car, Karen glanced longingly back at the dormitory. She wished she were still inside its secure, protective walls. Suddenly afraid, she realized that she was also outside the protection that her parents and friends could offer. She felt terribly alone and vulnerable, even with Jon there beside her.

The hospital waiting room was deserted except for six other abortion patients when Jon and Karen arrived. She recognized them as the same ones who'd attended the "orientation" the day before. The lack of other patients bothered Karen. *It's almost as though we're being isolated for some reason,* she thought. As she and Jon waited, her mind wandered. She imagined their little group of women as a leper colony, being forced to cry, "Unclean, unclean!" to anyone who passed their way.

She began to study the other women to guess their reasons for having abortions. She noticed that five of them had clustered in their own tiny clique at the far end of the waiting room. Karen suspected by the tight, short skirts and the heavy makeup they wore that they were all prostitutes.

Their voices carried clearly in the empty, quiet waiting room. Karen was appalled by their conversation as they nonchalantly discussed their previous abortions. Some of them had even relied on back-alley practitioners. Karen shuddered, thankful that a qualified doctor would care for her. *If abortion wasn't legal, I wouldn't be having one now,* she told herself.

The young women's voices intruded on her thoughts once more. Karen was shocked as she listened. "Just think how much money I'll be losing in the next two weeks!" the woman said, and the others glumly agreed.

Karen rebelled at the stigma of being placed in the company of prostitutes. But then she began to wonder how Jon saw her now. Was she dirty, profane, and prostituted in his eyes? She looked at the hardened, too-old faces of the five young women. The mark of sin showed clearly. Would her face change like theirs? Would people know by looking at her what she'd done?

She was glad when the only other abortion patient, a woman about thirty-five years of age, began talking to her. "I wish I knew whether I was doing the right thing," the lady confided. "For two cents I would call my husband and tell him to come and get me. I just can't decide if it's fair to bring a child into this world with the risk that the child will be deformed—fair for the child, I mean.

"I was exposed to German measles, you see. I'm willing to take the risk for myself. After all, the baby is part of me and my husband. We'd love it, but, I just don't know. Suppose the baby would have to spend its life in an institution? I don't think I could stand that, knowing I could have prevented it." She rambled on, telling Karen that she had three other children, paying no attention to the fact that Karen didn't answer. She only needed someone to listen.

"I have to go to work now, Karen," Jon said, interrupting the lady's monologue. "I'll pick you up as soon as I can." He kissed her quickly and left. "He acted as if he was glad to get out of here," Karen muttered. "I can't say that I blame him."

Just then her name was called by the receptionist. *Now what?* she thought as she went to answer the summons.

"Miss Blackburn, you need to fill out these papers. Apparently someone forgot to give them to you." The woman shoved the forms under the glass partition toward her. "Oh, and there's a question on your registration. Is your mother's name Sarah Blackburn?"

Startled, Karen answered, "Yes it is. Why?" Once again, she was afraid that they might contact her parents. *Will I ever lose that fear?* she asked herself.

"Oh, it's just a routine check of the records. Did you know you were born in this hospital?"

Karen didn't say anything. *No, I didn't know that my mother gave birth to me in this exact place . . . and now I'm going to abort my baby here.* The irony staggered her mind. *Given the same circumstances, would Mom have aborted me?* she wondered for a brief, shattering second, and then resolutely banished the thought. No sense going through the "what if's" again.

She stared down at the papers she had to sign. There was the one that cleared the hospital of liability in the event of her death. *Do women who have their babies sign this paper, too?* she wondered. After scrawling her name, Karen felt curiously as though she had just signed her life away. "How ridiculous!" she muttered.

The second form was from Welfare. It demanded that she repay the five hundred dollars whenever she became financially able. Would they send a bill or come knocking on her door someday?

When she asked the receptionist how they might collect her debt, the woman seemed irritated. "Just sign it if you want the abortion. It's a mandatory form," she stated impatiently. Karen signed it.

A nurse came into the waiting room just then, and led the abortion patients to their ward. Karen shivered as she quickly undressed and put on the scratchy white hospital gown that was provided. Then she crawled into bed and pulled the thin blankets over her.

As she waited for her turn, her fear grew. What would it really be like? Would she feel anything? Would she know when the fetus was taken? She wished Jon was there beside her, holding her hand. She felt terribly vulnerable in that alien environment.

If only I could talk to God, she thought in despair. *But I can't—not after everything I've done. I wonder if he still loves me. . . .*

She noticed a Gideon Bible on the table, and reached for it. She felt that she needed God at that moment more than she ever had in the past. "Or perhaps the truth is that I'm just now realizing how much I really do need you," she admitted with tears trickling down her face onto the pages of the Bible.

She turned to the Psalms, and the book fell open to the one hundred thirty-ninth chapter. The eighth verse leapt out at her, and lodged itself at the point of her need. "If I ascend up into heaven, thou art there: if I make my bed in hell, behold, thou art there." She stopped and pondered the thought for a moment and then read on. She skimmed the entire chapter, but kept returning in awe to the one verse.

"You're here, God!" she whispered in awe. "Are you really *here*—in this place? I find it so hard to believe." She trembled with relief as she remembered that his Word said, "I'll never leave you or forsake you." She felt his presence beside her and realized that her fear had gone.

A nurse approached her bedside and Karen smiled warily. Her eyes had focused on the ominous-looking needle the nurse held in her hand. "Don't worry," she said reassuringly. "This is the part that hurts most and it doesn't even hurt that bad. It'll help you relax." She gave Karen the injection.

Hot pain seared through Karen's arm. She blinked in surprise and forced back tears. "You lied," she flatly accused the nurse.

"Would I do that? Well, maybe a little, but from here on it's a breeze. You'll never feel a thing," she promised.

"I hope you're right." Karen listened to her footsteps padding quickly from the room and down the corridor. She gazed disinterestedly at the blank white walls and medical equipment that surrounded her and then shivered with a sudden chill. All hospital rooms are the same, she noted. Cold, sterile, impersonal. . . .

"I wish I were home," she cried, longing for an old patchwork quilt to warm her, her mother's arms to hold her, and her voice to say everything would be all right—that it wouldn't hurt too much, that she'd surely feel better in the morning. *But she isn't here—not in this place,* Karen thought, and again felt abandoned, with only a cold white sheet to comfort her.

"Oh, God," she prayed again, "Please help me! I don't want to feel anything. Even more than that, I don't want to *remember.* . . ."

The nurses wheeled her into the operating room and Karen lay there watching. The surgical team scurried about, rapidly blurring into neon-white images against the blackness that was enveloping her. But Karen was still conscious and listened intently to their chatter. "She's so tiny," one commented.

"Yes, and so young," another agreed, as they lifted her onto the operating table.

Their remarks irritated Karen. True, she was small, but after all, she was eighteen years old. "I can take care of myself," she muttered crossly, but no one paid any attention.

Moments later all her courage evaporated as another voice stated, "I think we're ready to begin."

"No, no!" she cried. "I'm still awake! Don't—"

The anesthesiologist clamped a rubber mask over her nose and mouth. "Breath deeply," he instructed her.

At first Karen wanted to gag on the sickly sweet gas, but as she relaxed she felt as though she were floating away from her body—separated from the event that was about to take place. . . .

"Where am I?" Karen mumbled as she tried to focus her drugged senses on the unfamiliar surroundings. The starkly furnished room and its antiseptic odor teased her memory. She frowned, trying hard to concentrate.

Then suddenly she felt chilled as she remembered where she was and why she was there. "I've just had an abortion," she whispered. The words sounded harsh to her ears and she half-way expected to cry. But no tears came. *I don't feel good, but I don't feel bad either,* she thought, somewhat surprised. *I guess I just feel blank—empty inside.*

For at that moment, Karen felt no inner pain or guilt over what she had done. Neither did she recollect any of her subconscious thoughts during the abortion. Instead, numbness like a pain-killing drug injection had enveloped her mind and spirit. *It's over.... It's over ... over ... over ...* her mind chanted as she drifted back to sleep.

Later she woke to find a doctor at her bedside. "Hi, young lady," he greeted her. "How do you feel?" His smile made her believe that he genuinely wanted to know.

So she thought for a moment, searching for the exact words to express how she felt. "Relieved, I guess," she answered finally. "I'm just glad that it's over."

He nodded. "Most women feel the same way. That's a good sign." He patted her shoulder and left the room.

But how do the other women feel? And why is being relieved such a good sign? Karen wanted to call after him, but instead she turned over and snuggled back under the covers. *I'm too tired to keep my eyes open, let alone think,* she admitted with a long yawn.

But before she could go back to sleep, a nurse came to take her temperature and blood pressure. "You're ready to be released," she told her.

So Karen dressed quickly and walked down to

the lobby. Jon was there waiting for her, his head buried in a textbook. As she approached him, she suddenly felt shy, almost afraid that he might reject her. "I'm ready to go, Jon," she said softly.

"Are you all right?" he asked, concern shadowing his smile. "How do you feel?"

"Actually, it didn't hurt at all," she answered. "And I feel just fine—normal, in fact."

"Good!" He looked relieved. "Then let's get out of here, OK?"

As they drove back to the college, Karen's mind kept churning. Jon seemed withdrawn, almost cold. Perhaps it was only her imagination. *Will the abortion make a difference in our relationship?* she wondered.

CHAPTER

9

In the weeks that followed, Jon and Karen began to argue over petty issues—something they had never done before the abortion. Everything they said or did seemed to be tainted by the experience.

When Jon asked her to type a term paper for him, Karen remarked irritably, "I'm not your slave. I may be your—" She dropped the sentence before she said the word on her mind, but the damage was already done.

"Forget it!" Jon shouted through gritted teeth. "I'll do it myself!" He grabbed the papers and slammed the door on his way out.

Karen felt miserably guilty as she recalled the incident. *He's such a lousy typist—he'll get a lower grade now because of it.*

Then she thought about breakfast that morning and groaned. Halfway through the meal, he'd reached over and speared one of her sausages. "That's mine!" she'd snapped.

"Well, excuse me! You never eat all of it, anyway. But I guess I should have asked before I touched anything that was yours." He glared at her. "And then I should have made sure that I didn't take it even if you said yes."

She didn't miss his innuendo but chose to ignore it. "I'm sorry, Jon," she apologized. "You're right. I'm not hungry at all. You can have it."

"No, thanks." Neither of them spoke again throughout the remainder of the meal.

Karen pondered that incident as well as others that had recently plagued their relationship as she sat studying in the college library. *Why do we have to fight about everything?* she asked herself. *Would everything be different if I hadn't gotten pregnant? Or if we'd never messed around with sex in the first place? Jon said it isn't the abortion that's the problem....* The words on the page kept running together. "I've read that paragraph three times!" she muttered, angry at her inability to concentrate on its meaning.

"Want to take a break?" Jon asked, pulling up a chair. "This place is so stuffy I thought a bit of fresh air might do us both good." Karen's eyes brightened as she noticed a smile on his face. Smiles seemed to be in short supply those days.

"Sure! I can't seem to get my brain to focus on this material, anyway." She hurriedly collected her notes and textbooks. The chair scraped noisily as she stood, provoking a frown from the librarian and several students. "Sorry," she whispered, trying to look properly apologetic as they left the room.

"Where to?" she asked him, hoping he wasn't planning to visit their favorite hideaway.

"There's a park with a playground that's not too far away. I thought we could use the swings and stuff. Sometimes I get that crazy feeling when it feels like spring is in the air—makes me feel young. . . ."

And innocent, Karen added silently, wishing it were only possible. "That'll be fun!" she agreed and slid into the front seat of the car.

Jon was right, she thought later, as he pushed her in the swing high up into the air. Her spirits soared. A fresh perspective. That's all they needed. She noticed a few tiny buds opening on the tree branches against the bright blue sky.

As Jon gently slowed her swing and brought it back to earth, she suddenly felt better about their relationship. "Give us a chance, Lord," she prayed. "Just give us another chance."

Jon held out his arms and Karen quickly responded. As he hugged her close, he murmured, "Karen, I do love you."

"I love you too, Jon." She reached up on tiptoe and kissed his cheek. "I just wish we could stop fighting and be the way we used to be— like we are right now."

A shadow crossed his face. "I don't know why we've been arguing so often. I hate it as much as you do," he admitted. "The only problem is, I don't think it can ever be the same. Too much has happened."

"What do you mean, Jon?" The sudden chill

she felt had nothing to do with the fact that the afternoon sun had begun to fade.

His face was glum. "I don't know, Karen. All I *do* know is that we can't go back and change the past."

"But can't we forget the past and start fresh? After all, nature does it once a year." She pointed to the new growth around them. "Can't we *forget?*" she repeated her question.

"Maybe you can, but I'm not sure *I* can." Jon's voice seemed agitated.

"Maybe you don't want to," she countered, noting his set jaw and bitter expression. "I get the feeling that you're trying to punish me for everything that's happened!" Karen fought against the feeling of hysteria that rose within her.

"That's not true. I'm not blaming you—it's just as much my fault, maybe more. I don't know what to *do* about it, that's all."

"Why don't you look forward, for a change?" Karen stormed, disgusted and angry with Jon's attitude. "Stop wallowing in the past!"

"It's no good, Karen." He sighed before continuing, "Everybody's noticed."

"Noticed *what?*"

"Us, what else? Some of my friends have said they think we ought to break up. They can tell we aren't happy."

"What business is it of theirs, anyway? How can we expect to work anything out if you're listening to them?"

"They're my friends, Karen."

"And I'm not?" Her eyes blazed angrily. "Is that what you're trying to say? What else did your 'friends' have to tell you?"

Jon hesitated for a moment and then replied, "They say you're bad news." He sighed, "It isn't easy to convince them otherwise. You've really been behaving like a brat."

"Thanks a lot." Karen's voice dripped sarcasm. "*You've* been a real prince—let me congratulate you." She thought about what he had just told her. *They say you're bad news,* echoed cruelly in her mind. "Do *you* think I'm bad news, Jon?" she asked him finally.

"I don't know, Karen. But I don't think you respect me anymore," he charged.

"Do you respect *me*?" she countered. "Answer me! Do you or don't you?" Her voice rose shrilly.

"No." His answer was flat, final.

"I guess it's mutual then!" She screamed the words at Jon, and then turned and ran blindly away. Trees, houses, streets all became an endless blur as Karen kept running with no destination in mind. "I won't go back—ever! I don't care if I ever see him again!" she sobbed, angry tears streaming down her face.

Then opposite thoughts intruded. *But I love him. I really do love Jon. I know we could make it work if he'd just try. Doesn't he love me at all?* She suddenly hoped that he had followed her, that once he caught up with her he'd hold her in his arms and tell her that he hadn't meant what he said.

Why do I always do such stupid things? she scolded herself. *I didn't really want to run away. All I want is for Jon to love me, to care what happens to me—to us.*

A sharp pain knifed her side, making it difficult to breathe. She stopped to rest and glanced behind her, half expecting to see Jon following her. But he was nowhere in sight, and despair gripped her. *He promised that he'd always love me, that he'd never leave me,* she thought bitterly. In her confused state of mind, she disregarded the fact that she was the one who'd left Jon behind.

Karen shivered as she looked at the unfamiliar street signs. *Where am I?* she suddenly wondered, noticing the sleazy businesses interspersed between ramshackle houses. Adult bookstores, massage parlors, and fortune-tellers blatantly advertised their wares. She fought a nauseous sensation as she gingerly stepped around piles of garbage strewn on the sidewalks. The twilight deepened, but no friendly streetlights twinkled to give her courage.

"Oh, Lord, please help me," she prayed over and over. She couldn't deny the fact that she was completely lost. Karen fought the rising fear within her as she finally located a telephone booth. It showed the ugly scars of repeated vandalism. "Now all I need is some change," she muttered as she searched her pockets, then searched them again, and yet one more time, but found them empty.

I can't cry—I can't panic! she told herself

desperately, but still the tears squeezed out from her tightly closed eyelids. She fought for self-control as she whispered to herself, "Stay calm, Karen, stay calm." She decided to knock at one of the houses and ask to use a phone, though none looked particularly welcoming.

Just then, she noticed a group of teenage boys approaching her, barely a block away. "Oh, Lord, help me!" she prayed again, and then turned and began to walk rapidly down a side street. "Don't let them follow me, God!" she cried, now running desperately through a maze of darkened streets.

Finally she saw a row of hedges bordering a city park. She glanced around, and seeing no evidence of anyone following, she ducked into a tiny alcove in the bushes. As she huddled there, she sobbed out her terror and bitterness toward Jon, blaming him for the predicament in which she found herself.

All at once Karen heard the ominous padding of heavy footsteps approaching her hiding place. She glanced about wildly, looking for a weapon to defend herself. Anything—a rock, a branch, a piece of glass—too late! As hands parted the branches that concealed her hiding place, a scream froze in Karen's throat, and suddenly the world was spinning, crazily going black. . . . She tried again to scream but no sound escaped her paralyzed throat.

"Karen, Karen! It's me, Jon!" He knelt beside her and gathered her in his arms, as he tried to calm her hysterical weeping. "I'm sorry, honey. I didn't mean to frighten you. Are you OK?"

"You really *did* follow me," she finally managed to say.

"Of course I followed you. I thought for a while that I'd lost you. Karen," she looked up and saw tears streaming down Jon's face, too. "Karen," he sobbed brokenly, "don't ever run away again. Promise me that."

She nodded and whispered, "I promise." She began crying again as she realized how badly she'd hurt and frightened Jon. "But how—how'd you know I was here?" she asked, puzzled because she hadn't seen him following her.

"I didn't know where you were," he admitted. "I had you in sight for a while, and then all of a sudden you disappeared." He buried his head in his hands, and spoke so softly that Karen could barely hear his words. "It got dark, and I just kept going. I prayed for God to show me where you were. I knew I had to find you—not just because you were lost, but because I love you. You believe me, don't you, Karen?"

She answered him with a hug, and he bent down to kiss her tenderly. "I didn't mean everything I said today—you know I love you, don't you?" He waited anxiously for her reply.

"Yes, I love you too, but—" she broke off as she recalled the ugly things that Jon had said. He'd said he didn't respect her. Her eyes brimmed with tears. What's love without respect? Would she ever be able to change the way he thought about her?

"Shh—" Jon put his finger lightly over her lips.

"We'll work out the rest of it," he reassured her. "I love you too much to lose you."

Another month passed. *But nothing's changed*, Karen thought bitterly. *What am I going to do?* she asked herself. Despite the fact that she and Jon claimed to love each other, their relationship hadn't improved. *All we do is fight*, Karen concluded miserably. *And what was it that Jon said last night? "Don't ask me to forgive and forget, Karen. That may seem simple to you, but I'm just not ready. Maybe the past is more real to me than it is to you."*

Karen felt angry and frustrated as she recalled his bitter words. Of course the past was real to her! she thought indignantly. After all, what had Jon gone through? She had forgiven him—why couldn't he forgive her?

"Thinking about Jon again?" Tricia asked, interrupting her thoughts. Karen nodded unwillingly as Tricia continued, "I know I should probably mind my own business, but we've been friends for a long time. I really hate to see you hurting like this." She hesitated for a long moment. "Why don't you break it up, Karen?" she advised. "You two are headed down a dead-end street. There *are* other guys on campus, in case you haven't noticed."

Karen chose not to answer and turned her face to the wall. She didn't want any other man, though at times she wasn't sure she wanted Jon, either. Of course she'd never admit that to Tricia.

"Are you sure you really love Jon?" Tricia continued. "I know you're engaged to him, but anyone could tell that you aren't happy." She paused for an answer, but Karen stubbornly remained silent. "Don't you want to talk about it?"

Karen stubbornly shook her head. "No, thanks, Trish," she answered. *If you only knew how much I need to talk to someone . . .* she admitted silently. Discouragement and loneliness overwhelmed her. She toyed with the notion of confiding her problems to her friend, and then dismissed the idea as both impractical and dangerous. She had not forgotten Mike's reaction to the abortion. *I'll never tell anyone,* she vowed once again. *No one would understand.*

Tricia shrugged at Karen's refusal, and then gave her a quick hug. "OK, but just remember that I'm available if you ever need a shoulder to cry on."

"Thanks." Karen managed a small smile.

Tricia collected her books and then paused, her hand on the doorknob. "Karen, maybe you and Jon *are* meant for each other," she acknowledged. "I don't know. Perhaps you just need some time apart to think things over. . . ." She left her thoughts dangling and closed the door softly behind her.

Karen felt outrage and confusion at the unasked-for-advice. At first she argued with Tricia's solution. Finally, Karen admitted the truth: Circumstances had changed. Disrespect and unforgiveness were two ugly dragons she hadn't counted on fighting.

She became aware of a song playing softly on

the radio. "Love means you never have to say you're sorry. . . ." She hummed the tune and contemplated the words. *Is love valid without forgiveness?* she wondered. *Don't people need to say that they're sorry? Can Jon really love me without forgiving me?*

She didn't want to answer the question, but the more she wrestled with it, the more firmly she believed Jon didn't love her—or if he did, that their relationship couldn't withstand his bitter, unforgiving attitude. "Tricia's right," she concluded. "If this marriage is meant to be, we should be happy. I still love Jon, but we can't go on this way."

A few minutes later, Karen stood waiting by the men's locker room door as Jon's P.E. class ended. He seemed surprised to see her. "What's up?" he asked, as they walked through the campus mall. When she didn't answer, he stopped and stared hard at her. "What's bothering you now?" he asked in a blunt, irritated manner.

How can I tell him? Karen wondered despairingly as her vision blurred with tears. She glanced around at the carefully landscaped campus, searching for a quiet place where they could talk. "Over there," she said finally, pointing to a secluded white wrought-iron bench surrounded by blossoming cherry trees. *In other circumstances this would be romantic,* she thought wryly as she sniffed the fragrant flowering buds.

But once they were seated, Karen found it no easier to begin explaining her decision. "I . . . I. . . ." She looked helplessly at Jon as she realized anew just how much she loved him. A lump rose in her throat, choking off her intended words.

But he was frowning, annoyance clearly etched on his face. "Quit playing games, Karen. Say what's on your mind." He ran his hand through his hair impatiently. "I have a lot of studying to do tonight. Midterms, remember?"

She took a deep, tremulous breath. "This isn't easy, Jon. . . ."

"Go on. I think I know what you're getting at."

She glanced warily at him. His voice had seemed strained, even a bit harsh. Yet his features were impassive, making her unsure of his reaction. *But if he knows what I'm getting at,* she thought. . . . "Then why don't you say it?" she suggested.

"You're the one who wanted to bring it up."

"All right!" she snapped. Jon could be so aggravating! "*I'll* say it then! I think we should break our engagement."

Her own words grated dissonantly on her ears, and she almost wished she could call them back. Then she reminded herself of the reasons why she was ending the engagement. In a quieter tone, she continued, "I love you, Jon, but love just isn't enough." She steeled herself not to cry, not wanting him to know how badly she was hurting.

"And what, then, is enough?" he asked quietly. She glanced at him and noted his stony expression. She wondered if he even cared to hear her response.

"Forgiveness and respect, Jon," she told him as

she slowly removed the engagement ring from her finger and returned it to him. "I don't think love can exist without them."

Tight-lipped, he took the ring and pocketed it. "Sorry," he said with a shrug, "Can't help you there." He stood up abruptly, and collected his books. Without another word, he left her sitting alone with her jumbled thoughts.

"He doesn't even love me!" she whispered in shocked disbelief. Only the whitened knuckles of her tightly clenched hands betrayed her desperate attempt at self-control as she watched him stride across the campus. With all her heart she wanted to beg him to stay. He hadn't bothered to discuss their relationship. Nor had he argued with her conclusions. For once, Karen had wanted to be wrong.

"Sorry," he'd said, and she felt as though he had slapped her with his mocking words. "If he loves me, then how could he say that?" She fought against the bitterness that threatened to overwhelm her. "I love him," she sobbed brokenly. "I don't care what he does. It won't make any difference to me—I'll still love him."

She suddenly shivered in the damp evening air. "I can't stay here all night," she mumbled, and began the long, lonely walk back to her dorm. Darkness and bone-chilling wind swept her soul as she began to realize how empty her world would be without Jon. She grew frightened as she contemplated it, never before realizing how much she had depended on him. "Oh, Lord," she prayed desperately, "please help us work this out. I love Jon so much."

But somehow, though she knew God could hear her prayer, she couldn't escape the nagging feeling that it had fallen flat. She felt no calm assurance that he would intervene in their situation. Instead, she felt uneasy, and her thoughts and emotions jangled discordantly. *But why?* she asked in despair and confusion.

The heavens seemed empty of answers.

CHAPTER

10

FOR several days, Karen refused to discuss her broken engagement. "Go away! Don't talk to me!" she wanted to scream at Tricia and the other girls. Finally they left her alone to brood about the past.

Karen felt unsure of her decision to end her relationship with Jon. *What if I'd only . . .* frequently plagued her mind. She found it impossible to eat, sleep, or study. Worse yet, her midterm exams were scheduled for the following week.

Bleary-eyed, she woke late Sunday morning, and was surprised to find Tricia there. "I thought you had gone to church," she commented.

Tricia shrugged. "Oh, I just thought I'd stay here and keep you company—that is, if you want any," she explained in an off-hand manner that belied her concern.

Karen scanned the morning newspaper, comprehending little of what she read. The headlines blurred as she found herself thinking about Jon again.

"Want to talk about it, Karen?" Tricia asked, noting her troubled expression.

Karen shook her head stubbornly. "I'm all right," she insisted. Then she felt Tricia's hand squeeze hers in an understanding, compassionate gesture. Her brave front abruptly shattered. "Oh, Trish, I don't think I can stand it! I love Jon so much," she sobbed bitterly.

"I know," Tricia consoled her. "But if God has chosen you two for each other, things will work out. Someday you'll have a stronger relationship. And if not . . . well then, isn't it better to find out now before it's too late?"

"But what if Jon doesn't do what God wants?" Karen argued, unable to accept what she felt were trite conclusions—certainly inapplicable to her situation. "What if we're supposed to be together and he decides he doesn't want me anymore?"

Tricia sighed. "I don't know all the answers, Karen," she admitted. "You'll just have to have faith that God is working for your best as well as Jon's in this situation, no matter how it turns out."

"I don't agree with that!" Karen exclaimed hotly. "How can I believe God is working for my best if he takes Jon away forever?" She tried to reconcile Tricia's words with her turbulent thoughts. *I can't even trust Jon to make the right decision, he's so mixed up!* she thought in dismay.

Her thoughts tumbled incoherently, and yet one kept stubbornly, inexorably surfacing. "I . . . I . . . ," she began hesitantly, and bit her lip to stop its trembling. "I don't think I can live without him," she confessed helplessly. "He's everything I ever wanted. I love him!" She stared at her tightly clenched hands in her lap.

Tricia glanced sharply at Karen, noting the fear and misery etched on her face. She took a deep breath as if carefully choosing her words. "That could be your main problem," she said quietly.

Karen wore a puzzled expression. "What do you mean?" she asked.

"The fact that your whole life centers on Jon," Tricia pointed out and then hesitated. "Look, I'll stop right now if you want me to. . . . I only want to help." Her face flushed with embarrassment. "I know that unasked-for advice is seldom appreciated."

"But I *want* to know what you think!" Karen insisted. "Maybe you have some answers for this mess—I know I don't." She unconsciously shredded a tissue as she reflected upon what Tricia had said. "Do you mean that I love Jon too much?" she asked disbelievingly. "I just don't see how that's possible!"

"No . . . and yes, Karen. You can't love anybody too much, unless you love him more than you love God."

"But—" Karen shook her head in consternation at the disquieting thought. "I love God. I always have!"

"Of course you do. But who do you love

more? Who's number one in your thoughts and decisions?" Tricia sighed deeply. "God has to be first. Your life just won't work any other way." She noted the stubborn, closed expression on Karen's face. "I can see that I've overstepped the boundaries," she commented with a sigh. "Maybe I'd better leave for a while." She threw a white sweater over her shoulders, and slipped quietly out the door.

Karen's mind whirled. Wasn't God first in her life? She'd just sort of taken it for granted that he was. She desperately wanted to hide from the issue. For a few moments, she felt angry with Tricia for even suggesting such a thing. "How dare she!" she sputtered silently. One of the first verses she'd ever learned was "Thou shalt love the Lord thy God with all thy heart, and with all thy soul, and with all thy mind." She knew that!

But do you really? probed a quiet voice deep inside her. *If you know it, do you follow it? Who really* is *number one to you, Karen?* The first commandment came unbidden to her mind: "Thou shalt have no other gods before me."

Karen's cheeks burned with shame. "You're right, Lord," she admitted finally. "I don't think you've ever been first—at least not in years. I considered myself first for a long time, then Jon became number one—my first priority, my first love. My idol," she whispered, shocked and sickened at the truth.

After spending a long, lonely day and a restless night, Karen rose early the next morning to talk to Tricia. "I'm sorry for the way I acted yesterday," she confessed, looking her friend straight in the eye. "You were right, of course, but how could I have been so blind?" She sighed bleakly. "I don't even know what to do about it. I know that I've done wrong, but I still love Jon just as much. I can't give him up! Do you think God would make me do that?" Karen's expression was horrified. Her desire to make God first place in her life was already weakening.

"Why don't you take it one step at a time?" Tricia suggested. "God understands—he *loves* you, Karen!"

"He couldn't!" Karen buried her face in her hands. "I feel so awful, so dirty . . . so wrong." She shuddered, hating herself for the faults she could so clearly see. "I don't think anyone, least of all God, could love me!"

Tricia hugged her. "I love you, Karen, and I know God loves you far more than I can. There isn't *anything* you could do that would cause him to stop loving you." She searched Karen's face, noting the spiritual hunger written there. "Would you like me to pray with you?" she offered.

Karen nodded. *What do I say?* she thought, suddenly panicking. A pastor's daughter was expected to pray well, and she'd had plenty of practice. She had even rehearsed her words during hymns to be ready in the event she were called upon. But Karen had no ready words for God this time. *Maybe Trish will pray instead*, she thought, but her hopes died as Tricia remained silent.

Finally Karen began, haltingly and with new humility. "Dear God, please forgive me for . . . for not making you first in my life. I was wrong to put Jon in your place. I'm sorry." She took a deep, shaking breath before continuing, "I want you to be the center of my life, Lord ... but you'll have to teach me."

Karen waited quietly, unable to find words to express her feelings and deep needs. The minutes ticked by, and still she waited—for what? She wasn't sure. And then she knew the reality of God's presence and peace as it surrounded, filled, and comforted her. "I love you, Lord," she whispered.

"Amen," Tricia finished and then hugged her. "Still friends?" she asked with a twinkle in her eyes.

"The best!" Karen declared. "Thank you, Trish." She frowned slightly. "I still don't know what to do about Jon, but—"

"One step at a time," Tricia finished the statement. "Let God handle it," she advised, glancing at her watch. She grabbed her books and headed for the door. "See you later. I've got a chemistry exam in five minutes!"

Karen stared open-mouthed as Tricia ran to class. "What a friend," she marveled. "She took time to help me with my problems—and right before a chemistry midterm, no less!" Karen knew, too, how difficult the class was for Tricia. "Please, God, clear her thoughts so that she can do well on the test," she prayed.

And I'd better get over to the library, she decided, collecting her own textbooks. *I have exams coming up, too.* Somehow, instead of feeling overwhelmed at the grueling task before her, she felt exhilarated. *I'm going to do well,* she decided, *because I want to. No more wasted brainpower!*

She felt more like herself than she had for a long time. *Karen, the studious one!* she thought, and giggled a little. *But no, I'm not even the old Karen,* she analyzed herself. *It's as though God is making me into my real self—the person he wants me to be.* She felt so happy, so whole inside that she half-skipped on the sidewalk, until a sobering thought struck her. *But will God include Jon in my life? Can I stand it if he doesn't?* She stood immobilized for a moment, and then resolutely climbed the library steps.

The hours passed almost unnoticed as Karen feverishly copied quotations from an enormous stack of books. She massaged her aching brow as she realized that she would have to type all night. Her report was due the following morning. She looked at her watch—only an hour until the library would close. "I have to finish this," she muttered. "I can't cart all these books home!"

A chair scraped noisily as someone sat down beside her. She glanced up. "Oh! Hi, Brad," she said. "I didn't even realize you were here!"

"Hi! Do you have time to talk for a few minutes?" he asked.

Karen was puzzled. What did Brad have to discuss with her? He was one of Jon's roommates, of course. She had always liked Brad. He had a zany, slightly crazy streak in him that could be both endearing and maddening. Karen frowned. She had never seen him in such a serious mood.

"What's wrong?" she asked nervously.

"That's what I'd like to know," he answered. "I'm concerned about Jon. The past few days have been the worst, but something has been eating at him for months. I want to help, but. . . ." Brad's gaze was penetrating, yet compassionate. "I care what happens to both of you," he emphasized. "Can you tell me what's going on?"

"You knew that we broke up—" Her words were half-question, half-statement.

"I figured as much, though Jon didn't say anything about it," he said. "Somehow I don't think that's the main problem. Is it?" He reached over and clasped her hand. She felt his strength and friendship. "I want to help," he repeated quietly and waited for her response.

The moments dragged by. Karen wanted to believe him. *I think I can trust him,* she tried to convince herself. Then her thoughts seesawed. *But if I tell him. . . .* "Oh, God, I have to talk to somebody! Will he act the same way that Mike did? I'm afraid, Lord—afraid that I'll never be able to trust anyone. . . ." She noticed that the library was nearly deserted.

"It's all right. Nobody can hear us," Brad said. "Go ahead, Karen. You can trust me. . . ."

Almost against her will, Karen found herself spilling out her story, her eyes glued to the library table. When she had finished, she hardly dared to look at Brad. *What will he say? What if he hates us like Mike does? Did I cause Jon to lose another friend? Oh, God, Jon will never forgive me—ever—if. . . .*

With great effort, she summoned her courage

and glanced up at Brad. She was amazed to see tears in his eyes. His shoulders slumped as though he were carrying a huge, invisible burden.

"If I'd only known," he repeated over and over. "Why didn't you and Jon tell me? I might have been able to help. I could have at least prayed for you." His expression was shocked and dismayed. "Some friend I am," he berated himself. "To think that you and Jon went through all that with nobody to talk to. . . ." He groaned deeply.

"Please don't feel that way, Brad," Karen cried. "It's not your fault that we didn't tell you anything. You've always been a good friend but—" She told him what had happened when they had foolishly confided in Mike.

Brad nodded. "That explains a lot of things," he said. "Mike's attitude toward Jon has really been rotten. I couldn't figure it out. Jon would just take it—he never fought back. It made me sick!" He remained silent for a moment, evidently reliving some of the scenes.

Then he continued, "But the important thing is that Jon needs our help. I don't know all the answers, but I do know that prayer works!" His smile was warm and accepting as he vowed, "I'm going to pray with you for Jon. God can straighten him out."

"Thanks, Brad. That's the best help you can give," she agreed. She noticed that the library was closing, and quickly gathered her papers and books.

"Let me carry those," he offered.

As they walked toward her dormitory, Karen mentioned how Tricia had helped her. "It feels so neat to have a right relationship with God," she confided to Brad. "I didn't realize how far I'd gone away from him."

She thought for a minute, trying to express the renewal that had taken place within her. "You've helped, too," she said, "more than you can imagine. You listened to me... and you cared." Her eyes filled with grateful tears. "Thanks, Brad," she whispered.

He set the books down on the step, and gave her a quick hug. "You and Jon will always be my friends," he assured her. "I love you both." Almost as an afterthought, he added, "You don't need to worry that I'll tell anyone, either. Your secret's safe with me."

Though Karen hadn't considered the possibility of gossip, she felt relieved to hear Brad's promise. She was thankful that she could trust him to keep her confidence. "Don't tell Jon, either," she begged. "At least, not for now." They stood on the doorstep and prayed for Jon.

Then as Brad turned to leave, he asked, "Are you going to the Spiritual Life Retreat next weekend?"

Karen gasped in surprise. *Could a year have passed already?* she wondered. "Of course I'll be there," she answered, and felt a quick stir of excitement. "I can hardly wait! What's the theme this year?" She remembered all too well what last year's theme had been!

Brad was already halfway down the street.

"But, God!" he called back to her and waved good-bye.

But, God? she thought in bewilderment as she unlocked the front door. *What does that mean?*

The days passed quickly as Karen took midterm examinations in all of her classes. "I think I did pretty well," she told Tricia, "but I'm glad this week is over!" She kicked off her shoes and flopped on her bed.

"Me, too!" Tricia agreed. "By the way, do you know whether or not Jon's going on the retreat?"

Karen shrugged. "I haven't heard," she replied. Her expression was thoughtful. "You know, Trish, before Jon and I broke up, I'd have never considered doing something if he didn't want to do it, too. But from now on, I've decided that I won't miss anything God has planned for me!" She began to carefully pack her suitcase, and her face became wistful. "I do hope Jon comes, though," she added softly.

Just then the intercom buzzed. *Who can that be?* Karen wondered as she went to the front door to answer it.

"Hi, Brad!" she greeted him. "We're almost ready, but aren't you a little bit early—say about an hour?"

"I'm not ready to go, either," he admitted. "But I thought you might want to hear some good news."

"What? Tell me!"

"Well," he drawled, "I just finished talking to Jon in the student lounge. Some of us managed to convince him to go on the retreat. How about *that*?"

"Fantastic!" Karen could scarcely contain herself. "Maybe the sermons will help him," she said hopefully.

"They'll probably help all of us," Brad pointed out as he turned to go. "I'll see you in a little while."

Later, when Brad pulled up to the apartment in his beat-up Chevy, Karen's eyes widened in surprise. *What's Jon doing in the backseat?* she thought angrily. She hadn't counted on his riding in the same car. *I'm not sitting with him!* She slid into the front seat next to Brad. Tricia rolled her eyes at the awkward situation and then climbed in beside her.

"One more to pick up," Brad informed them cheerfully. He drove up the block and stopped in front of Flanders Hall. An attractive blonde coed waited on the curb. Brad opened the rear car door for her to sit beside Jon. "This is Lisa," he said introducing her to them.

"Uh, oh," Tricia whispered to Karen. "I hope she isn't Brad's date! Maybe we should sit in back . . . ," she suggested hesitantly, but Karen acted as though she hadn't heard the suggestion.

Brad handled the wheel expertly as he drove in the rush-hour traffic. The car radio blared, drowning out the awkward silence. As he took the freeway off-ramp, Brad reached over and turned down the volume. He doggedly tried to engage the group in conversation, but his efforts met with little success. Karen remained silent, a half-smile on her face. *Serves you right,* she thought smugly, *for playing a trick like that on us!*

She felt immeasurably relieved when they arrived at the retreat center. As soon as the car was parked, Jon grabbed his suitcase and stomped away. They watched silently until he was out of sight.

Then Brad turned to Karen and apologized, "I'm sorry. When Jon said he'd go, he asked if he could ride in my car. I couldn't tell him that you were already coming with me or he would've changed his mind on the spot."

"And if you told me that he was going to ride with us, I would have stayed home," Karen finished the story for him. "No, *I'm* sorry! You were only trying to help both of us—and look at the thanks you got!"

Brad shrugged as if the fiasco didn't matter. "Aw, I suppose we all survived it," he said. He lifted their suitcases out of the trunk. "Where shall I take these?" he asked.

"Thanks, but we'll manage," Tricia said, grabbing hers as well as Karen's luggage. "Why don't you take Lisa's bags?" she suggested with twinkling eyes, Brad's ears turned crimson, and Karen and Tricia giggled all the way to their cabin.

"What a disaster!" Tricia chuckled, throwing herself on her cot. "Can you believe that trip?" she asked incredulously. "Jon in the backseat with Brad's date—at least I think she was! You sitting next to Brad. And me! I felt like Puck in *A Midsummer Night's Dream!*" They laughed hysterically at the incongruity of the situation.

"But, Trish, it isn't funny!" Karen protested in a mock-serious tone. Then they both dissolved into tears of helpless laughter again.

When they finally calmed down, Karen became thoughtful. "Trish," she said, "why was that funny? It didn't seem funny at all, but—" she shook her head in bewilderment.

"You goose!" Tricia smiled affectionately. "You just take life too seriously. Comedy and tragedy sometimes come in the same package," she explained. "It's all in how you look at it."

Karen moved busily about the small cabin, rearranging the meager furniture. "Not too cozy in here, is it?" she asked, and then giggled. "Of course it's all in how you look at it," she mimicked Tricia in a high, sing-song voice. A pillow connected with her head.

The pillow fight was so much fun that they almost missed dinner....

Karen thoroughly enjoyed the retreat. She spent much of her time sitting beside a tiny brook, her back against a sturdy tree, as she seriously explored her relationship with God. She wrote down Scripture references mentioned in the sermons, and then looked them up in her Bible. "Blessed is the man," she read, "who trusts in the Lord, whose confidence is in him. He will be like a tree planted by the water that sends out its roots by the stream. It does not fear when heat comes; its leaves are always green. It has no worries in a year of drought and never fails to bear fruit." "Oh, God," she prayed, "I want to be like that—to have that kind of confidence and trust in you, no matter what the circumstances are."

She struggled to grasp what was for her the most mind-boggling truth of all. "God wants to be your *enough*," the speaker had said. He challenged the students to make a list of everything that was important to them: "Your family, education, material needs and wants, job, life ambition, friends, a mate, personal freedom, health. . . ." Karen's list was long.

"Now imagine that all these things are gone. What would remain?" the speaker had asked. "God would! He wants you to love him and esteem his company so highly that if you had *nothing* else, you would be content to know him."

Do I love God that much? Is it fair for him to require that of me? Karen asked herself. *I think I could live without everything but the people I love. Could I be content to live without Jon—to even stay single—if that were God's plan for me? Is God my "enough"?*

"No," she admitted honestly. "But, God, I want you to be enough for me. Please do what you want with my life—and with Jon's, too. I'll trust you—even if it means losing him."

Karen had no way of knowing her future—no assurance that Jon would be her husband. Yet she was filled with a curious, inexplicable peace. It was the kind of peace that didn't let her down even when she saw him several times on the conference grounds.

Jon, on the other hand, had taken the retreat

to mean exactly that—he retreated farther and farther into his dark little world. She could read his moods, and keenly felt his unhappiness. Though she sympathized with his pain, she was determined that nothing, including him, would ever again interfere with her own personal growth. *My trust, my confidence is in the Lord,* she reminded herself.

As Karen waited for the final service to begin, she noticed that Jon was sitting in the pew just ahead of her, a little to the left. She surreptitiously watched him as he sat stone-faced through the service. She doubted that he was listening to the sermon. "Oh, God," she prayed, "can't you get through to him?"

Just then, a young woman stood up and interrupted the speaker. "I'm sorry," she apologized, "but I have to pray, and I can't wait any longer." As she stumbled toward the altar, the speaker abandoned his message and went to pray with her. Others followed in a steady stream—some alone, some in pairs.

Karen remained in her seat, pondering the meaning of the unusual occurrence. She watched as students prayed, and then asked forgiveness from others. Reconciliation seemed to be taking place everywhere. She suddenly realized the tremendous amount of power that was available. "The Holy Spirit is really here!" she whispered in awe and excitement.

A few moments later, Karen left her pew and knelt at the altar. As she began to pray, she felt someone's arm around her shoulders and realized that Brad had joined her. "I'm going to pray," she explained, "until Jon gives in and comes back to God."

"I'm going to be here doing the same thing," he answered. "And I don't care how long it takes."

Tricia came to kneel at Karen's other side. They prayed and wept for more than two hours, while Jon sat cemented to his seat, seemingly unaware that his friends were praying for him.

Suddenly Brad whispered, "He's here, Karen! Jon finally gave up!"

She looked across the room. "Where?" she whispered. "I don't see him. Are you sure?" Finally she spotted Jon. He seemed to be talking earnestly with the speaker. *What if Jon is telling him about our problems?* she worried. Then she felt ashamed. *Does it really matter if he does?* "I just want him to find help, Lord. If that's what it takes, it's all right with me." She glanced in Jon's direction again, and saw that he was praying. She thankfully continued her own prayer for him.

Another half hour passed before Jon finally stood. His eyes swept the room, and Karen was almost sure he was searching for her.

"Go on, Karen," Brad prodded. "He wants you. Anyone can tell that."

"I'm here, Jon," she whispered. Her heart was too full to wait any longer for him to find her, so she quietly walked over to him and slipped her hand into his.

He stood silently for a moment as he studied

her face. "Karen," he said finally in a choked voice, "will you forgive me for what I've done to you?"

"Of course, Jon. I forgave you a long time ago, remember? And I asked you to forgive me then, but you said you couldn't. Can you now?" *This is it,* Karen thought as she waited for that all-important answer.

"Yes, Karen," he responded earnestly. "God really talked to me about that. I asked him over and over to forgive me. He kept saying, 'Jon, I will forgive you, but you have to forgive Karen, too.' "

"I want to hear it," she pressed him. *I have to hear it,* she told herself.

Jon tenderly took her in his arms. With a shaking voice, he said, "Karen, I forgive you." She looked up at his face, and noted that his cloudy, stubborn countenance was completely changed. His expression glowed with a mixture of relief, joy, and peace.

Their friends had gathered around them, forming a circle of love. Jon shook his head in wonderment. "You'll never know how much I wanted to leave," he admitted. "I wanted to get up and run away, but I couldn't. Something held me here. . . ." He stopped to get control of his emotions before continuing. "I know it was your prayers." He paused and took a deep breath. "Thank you," he said humbly. "Thank you for being my friends . . . and for not giving up on me."

"Thank you, God, for getting through to Jon," Karen prayed silently. "It's worth it all to see him right with you—even if your plans for him might not include me." Did he love her enough to again ask her to marry him? Karen didn't know. Life held no guarantees. "God, you have to be my enough," she reaffirmed.

"I'm free!" Jon shouted exuberantly, startling everyone in the room. "I'm free!"

Karen smiled through her tears and saw that everyone in the room rejoiced with him.

CHAPTER

11

THE dormitory telephone rang shrilly from the far end of the hall. "I'll get it!" Karen shouted as she ran to answer it. *Could it be Jon?* she wondered. Though they had spent a lot of time talking since the retreat, he hadn't mentioned the subject of engagement or even asked her for a date.

"Hi, Karen." It was Jon! "I heard about a neat little coffeehouse today. Would you like to try it?" His question seemed a little hesitant, as if he weren't sure she'd say yes.

Would I? What a question! she thought, and then realized that he was still waiting for her answer. "Of course I'd like to go," she told him. "When?"

"I know it's short notice, but how about tonight—say about eight?"

That was in less than a hour! But Karen wasn't going to pass up the chance.

"I'll be ready! Bye." She hung up the receiver

and raced to her bedroom. She yanked the closet door open. There was no question about what she'd wear. She put on her light blue, full skirted voile dress, sprinkled with a tiny flowered print. A white bolero vest complemented the sheer long sleeves. Jon hadn't seen it yet, for she'd bought it on a shopping spree with Tricia and some other girls several weeks before.

Karen smiled as she remembered the fun they'd had. They had even gone into exclusive shops, pretending that they were planning a wedding. One would try on wedding gowns, while the others pretended to argue over bridesmaid's dress styles and colors. At first Karen objected to the scheme, but Tricia convinced her. "Go on, Karen," she said. "You be the bride this time. You're closer to the altar than any of us!"

At least I was then, Karen thought wryly, for at that time she and Jon had still been engaged. *But who knows? Maybe I will be wearing a wedding dress soon, after all. One can always hope!* She ran a brush through her waist-length brown hair, and willed the curls to behave themselves. Then she applied a soft rose lipstick and a last-minute dash of perfume. There! She was ready!

Tricia came into the room. "You look stunning!" she said. "All set?"

Karen nodded, but she suddenly felt jittery. She anxiously patted her hair and added a little more blush on cheeks that seemed too pale.

"Scared?" Tricia asked, and gave her an understanding hug. "Everything will be fine. I'll be praying for you," she promised.

The buzzer rang, but Karen stood frozen in front of the mirror. "Are you all right?" Tricia asked, quickly scanning her ashen face. "No, you aren't! Let's pray right now," she insisted. "Lord, please give Karen your peace this moment. Help her to trust you and remember that you're with her and Jon."

Karen took a deep breath. "Thanks, Tricia. I'm all right now," she insisted. "I just needed an extra shot of courage, I guess." She went to meet him.

Jon was waiting for her by the front door. "Ready?" he asked, smiling down at her. He offered his arm to her and they walked to his car.

They didn't talk much as they drove to the coffeehouse. What little they did say seemed stilted and shallow to Karen. *This isn't going to be easy,* she realized, noting that Jon was putting undue concentration on his driving, at least in her opinion.

The rich aroma of freshly roasted coffee beans greeted them as they entered the tiny establishment. Karen exclaimed over the antique coffee grinders and pots that served as decorations. The menu was complicated but fun to read. She finally chose Bavarian mint and Jon selected orange cappuccino.

As they relaxed with their dessert coffees, he finally broached the subject on both their minds. "I love you, Karen," he said, reaching across the table to hold her hand. "And I want to marry you."

"I love you, too, Jon." She hesitated. "There's just one thing. I . . . I want to know if we're starting over. Because if—well, I want things to be different this time."

He nodded. "I think I understand what you're saying," he said slowly. "I want God to be in control this time, and I want to start fresh—everything forgiven and forgotten. Is that what you mean?"

Her eyes sparkled with happy tears. "Yes, that's right. You really *do* understand! I want to go on from here ... to be free to marry you and love you ... to serve God together. It's not too late for that, is it?"

"No. We have God's forgiveness and our forgiveness of each other," he pointed out. "And he's forgotten what we did—the Bible promises that. Perhaps with time we can forget it, too." He placed her engagement ring in her hand. "Will you wear it?" he asked.

Karen had tears in her eyes as she put it on her finger. Then she looked at the ring more closely. "Jon," she said, "this isn't the same ring."

"I know. Do you like it?" he asked.

"Of course, It's. . . ." She searched for a word to adequately describe it. It's exquisite—but so was the other one."

"I know," he explained, "but I wanted us to have a brand-new start, so I chose this ring to symbolize it. It's a little smaller stone, but it's actually more valuable—"

"Thank you, Jon—I'll treasure it always," she told him softly, and then her thoughts spun on, leaving him behind.

"What are you thinking about?" he asked finally.

"Oh, it's hard to explain. I was thinking that maybe we'll be like this diamond someday." He looked at her questioningly. She struggled to explain the analogy. "Sometimes I feel as if I'm a smaller person, less valuable because of the things I did. But God can make my life count. Sometimes a smaller diamond reflects the light more beautifully than a large one does."

He nodded understandingly and squeezed her hand. "I know this much—I love you more now than I ever did before, and I expect our love to keep growing stronger and better."

Karen's eyes sparkled happily in the soft candlelight. "I love you, too," she whispered. "Everything will work out—I'm sure of it."

The months passed quickly as their love for each other deepened. There were so many important decisions to make. Jon would be graduating soon. Would he receive a call to pastor a church? If so, where? If not, then what? Seminary, perhaps? And Karen still had to plan their wedding.

She sat on a grassy hillside overlooking the campus. However, as she enjoyed the fresh air and soaked up the late May sunshine, she found it difficult to concentrate on European history. "It ought to be against the law," she grumbled, "to cram dusty old facts into my brain on a day like this!"

She rested her chin on her knees and daydreamed about Jon. He had changed so much, she realized. He was even a better student than he was before. Jon's grades had always been barely average, but since he had recommitted his life to God, he had applied new concentration and enthusiasm to his classwork. Karen felt sure that this term's report card would reflect his improved study habits.

Lucky Jon, she thought. His senior semester finals were already over, giving him a week to relax before graduation. Karen, as well as all other underclassmen, had examinations scheduled for the following week.

"Karen!" She glanced up and saw Jon charging up the hill, waving a piece of white paper in his hand. "It looks like a truce flag," she giggled, her mind full of battles and military strategies. "Thank God, at least *we're* not fighting anymore!" she said, closing her textbook with a smile.

"Look!" he shouted as he approached. "I made the dean's list!" He exuberantly scooped her up into his arms and hugged her tightly.

"Jon, that's fantastic!" she exclaimed, giving him a kiss. Then as he kissed her again more slowly and with greater passion, she felt a warm, familiar sensation inside her, which instantly melted her willpower. *Oh, Jon,* she thought, gazing up into his piercing, deep blue eyes, *you feel so good, so strong, so . . .* and then she grew alarmed as she read the sudden desire in Jon's face, too. She felt his body tense, and then he abruptly released her. She bit her quivering lip and stared at her tennis shoes.

"I'm sorry, Karen," he apologized with a dejected expression. "I guess it doesn't take much to get carried away."

"It's my fault, too," she said glumly. "It's just

so easy to get turned on. I wasn't even thinking about sex—"

"As soon as I had you in my arms, I was trying to think of a quiet, secluded place," Jon confessed. He looked at her appreciatively and commented, "You're a nice-looking temptation, you know."

"Thanks a lot!" Karen tried to glare at him but utterly failed. "You're a handsome temptation yourself," she pointed out. "But as you were saying before we *almost* got carried away, you had something to show me."

"Oh, yeah!" His face glowed with pride as he handed her the paper.

Karen scanned his report card. "All *A*'s and *B*'s—a three-point-five grade average! I knew you could do it!" she told him proudly.

"And that's not all!" he added. "I've had an offer to serve as youth minister in a church this summer!" He hesitated, and a shadow crossed his face. "The catch is that it's in Salem."

"Jon, that's wonderful!" she exclaimed, and then her face fell as the second part of his message dawned on her. *Salem?* she thought in dismay. *That's about two hundred fifty miles away!* "Of course I'll miss you ... we haven't even had time to plan our wedding yet." She sighed, thinking the situation over. "But it'll be the end of summer anyway before we can get married, and I guess I can take care of most of the details myself," she said, plainly unenthusiastic about the idea.

I can't be selfish, she scolded herself. *This is a wonderful chance for Jon. If only it weren't so*

161

far away! She tried to think of possible advantages that would outweigh the pain of separation.

Well, it would solve their problem with sex, she reasoned. But why, she wondered, did they have so much trouble stopping it when they knew they really wanted to wait until they were married?

She recalled the doctor's warning following the abortion. "You've already put your foot in the door," he'd said. "For your sake, keep some form of contraceptive handy." She and Jon had refused, feeling that they should depend on God as their source of strength.

Even so, they weren't one hundred percent successful. *Not that it's God's fault,* Karen thought ruefully. *We're so weak-willed sometimes. And the doctor was right about one thing,* she admitted. *It's a constant battle with temptation.* "I'll be so glad when we're finally married," she told Jon.

Jon nodded. "I know what you mean," he said. "I love you too much to risk losing your respect and love, Karen." He touched her face softly and shook his head. "It just isn't worth it," he concluded.

"But in the meantime," Karen added slowly, "as much as I'll miss you, I think that your job offer could be God's answer for us. Besides that, youth ministry is exactly what you want to do!" She fought to keep her tears back.

Jon's face lit up with eagerness and excitement. "Thanks, Karen," he said. "I hoped you'd see it that way. I didn't want to leave unless you were willing for me to go." He picked a long grass stem and chewed it reflectively. "What are you going to do this summer—besides plan our wedding?" he asked. "We've been so busy we haven't even discussed it!"

"Janie called just yesterday," Karen said. "She offered to let me stay with her and Larry this summer. I could walk to work from their house and save the bus fare. They'd just want me to pay my share of the groceries and watch the baby once in a while."

Jon thought for a minute. "Why would they do that?" he asked.

"I wondered about that, too," Karen admitted, "so I brought it up. Janie said that they really liked us both, and knew how difficult it was to scrape up money to get married. They just wanted to help, and figured that I could save the apartment rent by living with them for a few months. She said that she could use the company while Larry was working, and that I could help with housework and cooking if I wanted to—but that it wasn't necessary." Karen wrinkled her nose. "I suppose I should get all the practice I can before we get married," she said with an embarrassed blush. "I have a lot to learn." She keenly remembered the last disastrous meal she had prepared for Jon—raw baked potatoes and charred roast beef!

"You're just fine the way you are," he reassured her. "I have a lot to learn, too. I barely know what a hammer is!" They laughed, and then he said, "I think you should take Janie up on her offer."

"I already did," Karen said, glancing demurely at him.

"Oh." Jon seemed taken aback for a moment. Then he grinned at her and declared, "I'm marrying a woman who can make sound decisions!"

"Well, it wasn't anything like going two hundred fifty miles away," she pointed out. "I'd have talked to you first about something like that!"

"Whew! That's good to know!" he said in mock relief. "Well, we'd better get going. It must be close to dinnertime and I'm starved!" Holding hands, they strolled companionably down the hill.

After a light meal in the dining hall Jon decided to walk Karen back to her dorm so she could study.

"By the way," Karen said, frowning slightly, "I've been noticing that Tricia and Mark have been getting quite serious lately."

"What of it?" Jon shrugged. "Everybody gets serious this time of year. It's the weather," he explained.

"The weather? Baloney!" Karen didn't think much of his logic.

"Call it what you want," he said with a grin. "But getting back to the issue, why are you worried about Tricia? She and Mark haven't been dating that long."

Karen sighed. "I hope I'm wrong, but I think they're headed for trouble with sex."

"What makes you think that?"

"Oh, she's been coming in late, not talking much, looking a bit disheveled. She and Mark have been spending all their time together, and when they're in public, they act like they're alone. You know what I mean—touches, glances, kissing a lot.

"It's just that after the mistakes we've made," she continued, "it's easy to spot the signs. I remember when I used to see couples practically making love in public, I used to think, 'What do they do when they're alone?' Then I felt guilty for thinking that way. Now I realize that it's true. In most cases, people who behave like that are heading for trouble—if they aren't already there."

"Yeah, I've pretty much come to the same conclusion," Jon agreed. "What are you going to do about Tricia?"

"Is it my responsibility?" Karen asked, secretly hoping Jon would say no. She didn't relish the thought of confronting Tricia.

"Isn't it?" Jon shot back.

"Do you think I ought to tell her about us?"

"I don't think there's any other way to help her and Mark," he said. "I've noticed it, too, but I'm not close to either one of them. I doubt if they would appreciate my interference."

"All right, I'll talk to her the first chance I have," Karen resolved. "But I'd sure hate to lose her friendship, and if I happened to be wrong. . ."

"I don't think you are," Jon reassured her. "And I'll be praying. You can count on it." He bent his head to kiss her good-bye, and then she entered their room, wondering when and how she would talk to her friend.

She found Tricia carefully applying makeup. "You look terrific!" Karen complimented her and then asked, "Where are you and Mark going tonight?" She noticed that Tricia looked troubled at her question.

"I'm not sure yet," Tricia answered finally, and began rummaging in the closet.

"Lord, help me to say the right thing," Karen prayed silently. *Well, here goes—* she told herself bravely. "Do you have time to talk, Tricia?" she asked. "There's something I—I . . ." she fumbled for words.

"Sure, go ahead." Tricia glanced at her and looked puzzled. "Mark won't be here for at least a half hour," she said.

"You've always been such a good friend," Karen began hesitantly, "and there's something that's really been bothering me. I just don't know if I can say it. . . ."

"Why?"

"Because . . . I'm afraid that you won't be my friend if—" Karen buried her face in her hands and tears spilled through her fingers.

"Oh, Karen, there isn't *anything* you could say—or do—that would cause us to lose our friendship!" Tricia shook her head and smiled. "Go ahead and say it."

"OK." Karen took a deep, steadying breath. Then with downcast eyes and a voice that was frequently choked with tears, she told Tricia her story. She tried to explain why the tragedy had occurred. "We didn't plan for it to happen, Trish," she said, "but we made a lot of wrong choices."

Tricia sat on the bed with a stunned expression. "Dear God," Karen prayed silently, "did I misjudge the signs? Have I made a terrible mistake in telling her about everything?"

Then Tricia began to weep. "Oh, Karen," she cried, "why didn't you let me know before now? I wish I could've helped you. I would have, you know." She stopped and sighed, as if she knew that the past couldn't be changed. "But thank you for telling me."

Tricia looked away as she confessed, "Mark and I almost blew it the other night. We've been so tempted." She glanced quickly at Karen's face, reading her reaction. "You knew, didn't you?" Her question was almost a statement. "That's why you said all this, wasn't it? Or did you tell me because you needed to get it off your chest?"

Karen's expression was compassionate. "I didn't need to tell anyone for my sake—not now, anyway," she answered. "But once a person's been involved sexually, it's easy to see when others are heading in the same direction. I care about you and Mark, and yet I didn't want to say anything about what I *thought* was happening in case I was wrong."

"I never thought it could happen to either of us," Tricia said almost disbelievingly. "But if it happened to you . . . I know I'm not any different or better." She hugged Karen then, and they cried together.

"And as for the abortion," Tricia continued, "my own family's been facing the question. My older sister is married, with four children. She just found out she's expecting another one. Her

167

health isn't good, and she barely has the strength to take care of the ones they already have. They're Christians, too, and they're mixed up about what to do."

"I don't know the answer for them," Karen said. "All I know is that it was an awful experience that I'd like to leave in the past."

"But what about now, Karen?" Tricia asked. "Do you and Jon still have problems with sex? I need to know the truth, because I'm wondering if there's any hope for Mark and me. We've already gone pretty far. . . ."

Karen thought carefully about her answer. She had to be honest. "It's not easy," she said finally. "In fact, it's next to impossible to stop having sex once you've begun—without God's help, that is. Even so, Jon and I have a tough time." She looked levelly at her friend before continuing. "I don't want to kid you about how hard it is, but there is hope—it's called prevention."

"You're using contraceptives?" Tricia was shocked.

"No!" Karen shook her head. "*Prevention* as in no parking, staying away from secluded, romantic areas, and no dates without a destination and planned activity. But on the plus side, we have a half hour devotional time together each day, and we do something special with friends each week. We've also been attending all the college activities, and we're spending time just developing our friendship and planning our future." She smiled slightly. "Have you noticed us doing any of that, Trish?"

"Now that you mention it, yes! But I didn't

think too much about it, because I'd gotten so wrapped up in Mark." She blushed furiously. "I can only guess at what you went through," she admitted, "but I know how miserable and guilty I've felt lately. You know what, Karen? I can't believe how silly I must have sounded to God, asking him if it would be all right to have sex since Mark and I have fallen in love!"

"Believe me, he's heard the story before," Karen remarked dryly.

"Well, this is one story that's going to change right now, before it's too late!" Tricia resolved firmly. "*We're* going to set up some rules, too." She squeezed Karen's hand. "I have an idea of how hard this was for you to tell me," she said, "and I want to thank you for being a friend—a *real* friend."

"You're welcome," Karen responded softly. "If I helped, it was worth it."

CHAPTER

12

KAREN could hardly contain her pride as she watched Jon stride eagerly across the platform to receive his diploma. *Another goal accomplished,* she thought a trifle sadly, for she knew they'd miss the college. She had decided she wouldn't return after they were married. Maybe someday, though. But then she began to daydream about their wedding plans. Her thoughts were far away as the graduation speakers droned on endlessly in the muggy auditorium.

Afterwards, she quickly found Jon and hugged him. "I'm so proud of you!" she whispered. Then his family gathered around them, and Karen tried to cope with the bewildering introductions. She was thankful that Jon had already shown her pictures of his parents and siblings on both sides of his family. Even so, she was confused, for his uncles, aunts, cousins, and grandparents had also attended the graduation.

Jon's family seemed to be excited about the upcoming wedding. His parents were warm and friendly to Karen, which she couldn't help contrasting with her own parents' view of Jon. *Oh well,* she thought philosophically. *They'll come around. It'll just take time.* She had to admit that her parents' letters seemed warmer lately, and they had included Jon at the end of the last one. "Give Jon our love and best wishes on graduating," they'd said.

The day after graduation, Jon helped Karen move into Larry and Janie's home. He carried her small pile of belongings into the house, and then stood beside his car talking with her. "Do you realize," he pointed out, "that all you have is a couple of suitcases and three boxes? I think I have even less than that. How are we supposed to fill up a whole house?"

"Let's see," she replied. "We'll put your guitar in one corner and the stereo in the other! There! Instant home decorating in one easy lesson!" They laughed and then Karen said, "We need so many things that I hardly know where to begin."

Jon grinned. "Wait until after the wedding," he advised. "Then we'll know what we still need."

"Jon! That isn't why you ask people to come!" Karen said indignantly.

He shrugged and grinned. "I know, but it's true. Look how many presents we've bought for everybody that had the good sense to get married in June!" Noting her shocked expression, he became serious. "I was mostly teasing, Karen. But you know the custom—and it's a good one.

People like to share a happy occasion, and most newlyweds need all the help they can get." He shook his head. "I know we do."

Karen smiled impishly at him. "Don't forget the showers."

"Showers?" His expression was puzzled.

"Tricia's giving one for me next week," Karen told him. "It's a lingerie party." She giggled as she saw Jon's red face. Still, he looked pleased. "And," she continued, "the ladies in my home church are giving me a kitchen shower right before the wedding. Mom wrote about it in her last letter." She looked homesick for a moment. Then she thought about Jon's departure and began to cry. "I don't think I'll be able to stand being here without you," she said, burying her head in his chest.

"You'll make it, Karen," he said, trying to comfort her. "Time will go faster than you think, and before you know it, we'll be married!" As he hugged her closely to him, he confessed, "I'll miss you, too, though. It won't be easy for me, either. But I'll call," he promised, "and I'll write once a week."

"That'll be the day!" Karen said disbelievingly. She remembered just how often Jon had written during their last separation. She smiled tremulously and said, "I hate to say good-bye, but I know you have to get on the road. It's a long trip."

He sighed and tenderly smoothed her hair. "Bye, Karen—for the last time." He kissed her, and then got into his car. "After this, we'll be together for the rest of our lives!"

She stood waving and smiling through her tears until he was out of sight. Then she squared her shoulders and went into the house to unpack.

"Do you mind staying in the baby's room, Karen?" Janie asked. "She sleeps all night now, so she shouldn't disturb you."

"No, of course not," she answered. "Anna's a little dear. Besides that, she's one roommate that can't argue with me—yet, that is!"

The weeks did, in fact, pass quickly as Karen worked full time in the coffee shop. When she wasn't working, she tried to help Janie at home. "Let me do that ironing," she insisted. "You need to rest. Here," she said, pulling up a chair. "You sit right here and chat if you like while I whip through these. It'll go faster that way."

Janie gladly obeyed. With her feet up on a stool, she asked, "How's Jon doing? I've noticed that he writes often."

"Yes, he does," Karen agreed, as she sprinkled one of Larry's white shirts. "He's busy and loves youth ministry." She looked concerned as she said, "I just wish I knew what we're going to do come September. He only has a summer job. Of course," Karen added, "I have my job. We can make it for a while on that if we have to."

"It'll all work out," Janie said confidently. "Have you decided on wedding colors?" she asked.

"Yes, I think so," Karen answered. "I think Tricia would look nice in lavender. But I don't know what to do about the men's tuxedos. What do you think?"

"I don't know—they can always wear white jackets and black slacks. Aren't I original?" Janie wrinkled her nose and laughed. "Of course, you *could* try to make them wear lavender shirts, but you might have a revolt on your hands!"

The telephone rang and Janie reached for it. After a moment, she said, "It's for you, Karen."

Karen eagerly took the receiver. "Hello?"

"Karen?" Jon's voice seemed so far away. "Are you ready for some good news?"

"Yes! What is it?"

"The church has offered me a full-time job as associate pastor starting in September! How would you like to move to Salem?"

"Oh, Jon!" Karen sat down weakly.

"You could transfer your credits to a school down here if you wanted to finish," he pointed out. "And they've offered to let us live in the parsonage as part of my salary. The pastor bought his own home last year, and it's sitting empty.... Karen? Karen, are you there?" Jon shouted over the telephone line.

"Yes, Jon, I'm here. I'm just in shock! It's wonderful! What a surprise!" she exclaimed. "Of course I'll move to Salem!" The phone call was a luxury, and so they quickly ended their conversation. But the glow stayed with her for days.

Karen had little time to think about her past. She was too busy shopping for her wedding dress, ordering invitations, choosing music—and to bring her down to earth, taking orders and serving food at the coffee shop.

Late one evening, after working ten hectic hours, she came into the house and kicked her shoes off. She collapsed onto the sofa, and idly picked up a magazine to read. She glanced at the cover, and then stared horror-stricken at the photo—a full-color picture of a human fetus in a laboratory jar. She flung the magazine across the room and began to scream hysterically.

Janie came running, pulling on a housecoat. "Karen! Stop it!" she cried. Finally in desperation, she slapped her face several times. At last, Karen calmed down and sobbed quietly on Janie's shoulder. "Karen, what is the matter?" Janie asked over and over, but Karen could only cry, too terrified to tell her.

After several minutes, Janie noticed the magazine on the floor. She quietly went over and picked it up. "Does it have anything to do with this?" she asked, pointing to the horrible picture.

"Yes," Karen whispered, and began to sob again. Under the circumstances, she knew she had to explain what had happened. *Will they throw me out of the house? Where will I go?* Karen wondered, and fresh despair overwhelmed her.

Perhaps Larry and Janie would tell the church. Jon would get fired! And if that happened, other churches would find out! He'd never be a pastor then. Her mind leaped ahead to all sorts of catastrophic conclusions.

"Tell me about it," Janie prompted in a kindly tone. Karen tried to explain what had happened to her and Jon, but she was incoherent much of the time. Janie worked hard to understand her story.

"Listen to me, Karen," she said firmly when Karen had finished. "Larry and I already knew that you and Jon have been sexually involved."

"But how?" Karen gasped, her face ashen. "How could you have known?"

"Remember the church picnic?" Janie asked, and Karen nodded. "You were sitting with a bunch of married women," she reminded her, "and we were sort of talking about sex—you know, birth control and all that. Paula even made a little joke." Karen nodded again and smiled a little.

Janie smiled, too. "It was funny, wasn't it?" Then she continued, "I just noticed that you seemed to understand quite a bit of what the ladies were saying—more than what a sexually naive person would comprehend."

Karen was aghast. "Does *everybody* know about us?" she asked.

"Oh, I sincerely doubt it," Janie tried to reassure her. "Not everyone has that kind of radar equipment."

Like Jon and me, Karen thought. She suddenly realized that if they could pick up signals from Mark and Tricia, then other people could have a pretty fair idea of what Jon and she had done. *Maybe that's why my parents were so suspicious of our relationship,* she thought. *I don't think we fooled them for a minute.*

"Karen?" Janie was trying to gain her attention. "I have something that I want to tell you," she said. "No matter what you've done, Larry and I could never condemn you." She bit her lip ner-

vously. "You see, Larry and I had to get married—
and then we lost the baby before it was born.
We love each other and the Lord, too, but. . . ."
Tears came to Janie's eyes as she continued,
"After all this time, the problem that we faced
then—five years ago—has been awfully rough
on our marriage. We've learned some hard les-
sons. That's one of the reasons we asked you to
stay in our home. We love both of you, and we
want to help if we can."

Karen was silent for a long time as she tried to
sort out their conversation. Finally she spoke.
"All right, Janie, I can understand what you're
saying, but. . . ." Karen wanted to argue but she
wasn't sure how to phrase it. She tried again.
"Janie, I had an abortion. I think that's worse
than what you did—isn't it?" Karen wasn't sure,
but somehow an abortion seemed worse.

"In whose book?" Janie retorted. "Listen, you
know as well as I do that God doesn't rate sin
on a scale of one to ten. It's all the same to him.
You've asked his forgiveness, haven't you,
Karen?"

"Yes, but it's hard for me to believe that he
forgives me."

"*Forgave*, Karen," Janie corrected her. "And
forgot. Don't leave out that part. Everytime you
bring it up to God, he says, 'Huh?' He doesn't
even remember your sins."

Karen nodded. "OK, I can agree with you on
that, but I know the church doesn't look at it
that way. I don't think they would forgive us—
or forget, for that matter. And I don't think my

folks could, either. At the very least, I think they'd hate Jon, and I couldn't bear that." She covered her face with her hands, and her words were taut with pain. "I love them all, Janie—my parents and Jon. I don't think I could stand in the middle between them," she cried. "I don't dare ever let them find out!"

Janie wore a determined look as she stated. "Look, Karen, the Bible says that we are to forgive one another as Christ has forgiven us. If the church and your family can't obey that, whose problem is it?"

"Mine," Karen insisted stubbornly.

"Karen! It's theirs, and you know it." Janie was firm. Then her tone softened. "Let's talk to the Lord about it, Karen," she suggested. She prayed then, asking God to begin healing Karen's subconscious thoughts—all the horror that was buried deep in her memory.

"You'll always have scars, Karen, but you'll eventually heal," Janie assured her. "And someday," she smiled at her affectionately, "maybe those scars will urge you to help someone else."

Karen picked up the magazine and looked again at the cover. "Do you think that—" she found it hard to express her thoughts. *What do I call this?* she wondered. *This is a baby, a boy.* The picture continued to horrify her with its implications.

"Do I think what, Karen?"

Karen's thoughts were confused. *I can't say our baby, or him or her . . . yet fetus seems all wrong, too.* She struggled with her question. "Do you think that . . . it . . . looked like this?" she asked finally. Her forehead beaded with sweat at the awful thought.

Janie frowned. "What did they tell you? How far along did you say you were?"

"Eight weeks."

"No, Karen," Janie said, shaking her head, "I don't think it looked like this."

Karen felt immeasurably relieved. "That's good," she said, "I wouldn't have done it, if. . . ." She left the rest unsaid.

"I know," Janie said softly, and followed Karen into the baby's room. Anna stirred, and Janie carefully tucked the blanket around her.

"She's so precious," Karen whispered, and was surprised at the yearning that stirred within her.

CHAPTER
13

KAREN swatted blindly at the alarm clock. "Five o'clock?" she grumbled. "Who set it for that unearthly hour?" She groaned and pulled the covers over her head. A few minutes later she sat bolt upright—"Today's my wedding!" she exclaimed.

She jumped out of bed and threw on a pair of jeans and a T-shirt. "So much to get done," Karen muttered, scattering papers everywhere as she searched for her list. "Ah, here it is," she said, and sat on her bed to read it over. "Pack suitcases, breakfast at six with Mom and Dad, hair appointment at seven, pick up cake at eight-thirty, be at the church at nine, and then wedding begins at ten." She glanced at the clock. "Five fifteen? I'll never be ready in time!" she cried, and raced for the shower.

But at nine-thirty that morning, Karen was posing for some prewedding pictures. "You look absolutely beautiful!" her mother said proudly, adjusting her veil and train. All too soon, the knock at the door signaled that it was time to begin.

Karen stood with her father at the entrance to the sanctuary as the organ began to quietly play the wedding march. She watched soberly as Tricia walked down the aisle. Then the organ swelled and the audience stood. Karen took her father's arm and stole a quick glance at him. He smiled broadly at her and his eyes twinkled. "Let's go, Karen!" he whispered. She nodded in return, and a lump came to her throat.

As they walked slowly toward the altar, she noticed the morning sunshine filtering through the stained-glass windows, the faces of friends and family, the highly polished wooden pews, and the beautiful pink and lavender floral arrangements. Then she saw Jon waiting patiently for her, and read the love and pride reflected in his eyes. *Oh, Jon!* she thought, *I love you!*

"Who gives this woman to be married to this man?" the minister's words rang out, calling Karen to attention.

"Her mother and I do," Karen's father said firmly, and as he gave her arm to Jon, she knew that her parents were relinquishing all rights. They were trusting Jon to care for her.

She smiled up at Jon as they promised to love and cherish each other forever, regardless of circumstances. As they knelt to dedicate their marriage to God, Karen prayed silently, "Thank you, Lord, for giving Jon to me—and for holding us together through the hard times we've already faced. Be our guide. . . ."

She felt Jon's strong hand on her arm, helping her to rise and face the congregation. The minister announced, "May I present to you, Mr. and Mrs. Jon Hamilton!" As Jon lifted Karen's veil and kissed her, she felt so different! They were finally married!

After the reception, Jon and Karen packed their wedding gifts into the car, and set off for their new home. They planned to move into the parsonage, and then spend the remainder of their honeymoon camping at Crater Lake.

They pulled up in front of their first house early that same evening. "Well, how do you like it?" Jon asked, scanning her face for clues.

Karen eagerly jumped out of the car. She noticed the carefully landscaped yard, the neat white picket fence, and the dark red freshly painted cottage, trimmed with white shutters. "It looks so cozy!" she exclaimed, and pointed out the brick chimney that perched on top the wood-shaked roof. "Is there a fireplace?" she asked. "Hurry, Jon! Where's the key? I want to see inside!"

Jon stalled for a moment to tease her. He had an amused expression on his face as he noted her impatience. Then he unlocked the door, picked her up, and carried her over the threshold. "Welcome to your new home, Mrs. Hamilton!" he said, and kissed her before he set her down.

"Hardwood floors! How beautiful!" She scurried about, exclaiming over each room while Jon carried in their belongings. Then he built a small fire in the fireplace, and Karen sighed romantically. "A wedding, a husband, and a home—all in one day!" she said. "Pinch me! Is this real?"

"They say that after every wedding comes marriage," Jon pointed out as they sat on the living room floor and roasted hot dogs for dinner. The real challenge had begun—the process of becoming one. . . .

Several months later, Karen found herself sitting by the living room window, staring at the rain-splattered glass. Jon was gone *again*, and she felt lonely and frustrated. It seemed that church committee meetings, visitation, office hours, youth activities, and regular services consumed every minute of his day. "The only time I ever see you is to sleep and eat!" she'd complained that morning.

"I thought you were an expert on living in a pastor's family!" he shot back bitterly. "I can't help it, Karen. I'm not the boss. Pastor Blake says I have to be at the board meeting at seven. I'm not God—I can't be two places at once! Will you get off my back?" He slammed the door as he left.

Marriage sure isn't what it's cracked up to be! Karen reflected. *We thought we'd be able to spend more time together, but it's worse now. And it's not Jon's fault, either,* she admitted to herself. *I guess I shouldn't have griped. I know he wants to be with me, but he's caught in the middle.*

She poured another cup of coffee and noted the time. She'd have to leave for work in another hour. Though Karen was thankful that she'd found a job as a waitress only eight blocks away, she found herself resenting the low pay for the backbreaking labor. Then, too, whenever Jon *did* have a chance to be home, more often than not she was at work. *This business of becoming one is the pits,* she thought, feeling utterly defeated. *Everything seems to pull us apart—our jobs, finances, even sex.*

Karen couldn't figure it out. She'd read magazine articles that had advocated premarital sex. "Try it out first," the writers advised, "then you'll know if you're sexually compatible. Why risk a shock after you're married?" The idea seemed reasonable. *Not that they had been "testing compatibility,"* Karen thought with a bit of wry humor. Still, she had been certain that sex would be one area that she and Jon wouldn't worry about once they were married.

Ironically, they soon discovered that premarital sex had actually *created* hang-ups in their relationship. *Take last night for example,* Karen thought, and her mouth compressed into a thin, hard line as she remembered.

"What's wrong with you, Karen?" Jon had asked. "Or is it me? Don't you love me?" Sex was a difficult, explosive subject for them to discuss.

"I don't know what's the matter, Jon," she'd sobbed, knowing that her lack of desire wasn't normal—especially not for a new bride. And yet, she wasn't about to take all the blame. She often felt that Jon was merely using her for his own sexual gratification. "Don't you love *me*?" she had thrown the question back at him.

But why did I enjoy sex so much before we were married? Her untouched coffee became cold as she sought the elusive solution to their problem. The minutes ticked by. Karen retraced the steps of their relationship.

Shamefaced, she truthfully answered her own question. *I did it because I enjoyed the excitement and the danger,* she finally admitted. *But now that we don't have to worry about being found out or having an unwanted pregnancy, I'm ... bored. What an awful word,* she told herself. *What happened to our love?*

Sex never was a real expression of love for either of us! she suddenly realized. She had blamed Jon for "using" her body, for lusting instead of loving her as a total individual. She felt deeply ashamed as she admitted to herself that she had also used Jon. *No wonder God said no,* she thought as she finally recognized the damage that their premarital intimacy had caused. Once Karen understood the root of the problem, she asked God to change her wrong attitudes toward Jon in that area.

"I want to really love you, Jon," she told him later that evening with tears in her eyes. "I want us to be one—the way God intended."

"I love you, too," he said, holding her close. "We are one, Karen. And at the same time, we are *becoming* one. It's a process, a goal—something to work toward." He kissed her gently and asked, "How would you like a mini-vacation?"

"When? Where?" Karen was ready to pack the suitcases!

"There's a pastors' and wives' retreat next week, and the church is paying our way. We'll have lots of time by ourselves—which we need—and some workshops, too. Do you want to go?" He smiled, reading the answer on her face. "By the way," he added, "I already squared it with your boss."

Karen could hardly wait. Imagine, a whole week with Jon with no telephone calls, committee meetings, or other interruptions! It seemed more like a honeymoon than the one they'd had.

The following Monday found Jon and Karen in their own private cabin in the woods. "It's rustic," she said, glancing at the pot-bellied stove and the heavy patchwork quilt on the bed. She noticed a lantern on the table, and several candles lying on the scarred antique dresser. "No electricity?" she asked.

"It's rustic!" Jon replied, laughing.

During the week, Karen enjoyed the time she spent with Jon. They took long hikes through the woods, and canoed on the lake. Sometimes they talked; other times they were content to sit silently, enjoying each other's nearness.

The workshops were fun, too, Karen discovered. One day she chose to attend a special conference just for the wives. The leader was already talking when Karen arrived, so she found a chair in the back and began to listen.

"We all have burdens," the leader said, "and they're like little wrapped boxes that we've given to God to handle." She smiled at the women. "And do you know what? We're forever being Indian givers! What do you have in that little box that you keep grabbing back from God?" she asked.

Karen didn't have to think very hard on that question. Lately, she had pulled the lid open on her personal Pandora's box and had rummaged through its contents. Those old, horrible memories. . . . If only she hadn't. . . .

The leader spoke again. "Now, close your eyes and picture Christ coming toward you, and you have that little box cupped securely in your hands. What is he saying to you?"

Karen obediently closed her eyes. The picture of Christ immediately became so vivid—the colors so brightly hued and his form so dazzling—that she felt she was physically in his presence. As he walked toward Karen in her mind, she ran into his outstretched arms. She felt herself shedding bitter tears as he said, "Karen, I love you." Just four simple words, but she felt the message was addressed specifically to her. It was as if he would have died just for her if she were the only one who had ever sinned, she realized. The thought staggered her.

Then Christ spoke again. "Karen, you gave me the box before. I forgave you and forgot about your sin, but you've taken it back again because you haven't forgiven yourself." He waited as she pondered his words. Then he asked, "Karen, for your sake, will you forgive yourself?" She nodded, and he reached for her tattered little sin-box, turned, and flung it into the sparkling sea behind him.

It's gone forever! she realized, and her spirit felt light and clean and free. The old heaviness had vanished. *I thought I'd always have to live with my guilt, because it never really went away,* she thought in amazement. *No one ever told me that I had to forgive myself!*

CHAPTER

14

"GUESS what, Jon?" Karen smiled at him across the kitchen table. "I love you and I'm so glad we're married."

"Same here—but is that supposed to be a big secret?" He laughed and kissed her hand. "It's been a wonderful two years, I'll have to admit," he said. "Happy anniversary!"

Her eyes danced merrily. "I do have a secret, though," she said. "Guess what?"

"Hmmm. . . ." He pretended to think hard. "We won the magazine sweepstakes and we'll be independently wealthy for the rest of our lives!"

"No, independently poor is probably more like it—I'm pregnant, Jon!" She looked anxiously at him, hoping that he'd be pleased.

She needn't have worried, for Jon, though he sat dumbfounded for a moment, grinned with delight. "Wow! That's great, honey!" He kissed her as though she were fragile enough to break.

They lay awake for hours that night, planning their baby's birth. Karen had already mentally decorated the nursery. She'd priced cribs and baby clothes. She'd even discussed the financial arrangements with her doctor.

"What shall we call him—or her?" Jon asked sleepily. "Have you thought of a name? You've covered all the other bases!"

"I wonder," Karen thought aloud, "when 'it' becomes a boy or girl. . . ."

Karen was three months pregnant when she miscarried the baby. Her doctor called it a "spontaneous abortion." The term made Karen angry. It seemed to point a finger at her as if the miscarriage were her fault. She mourned the baby, and there was nothing Jon could do to relieve her depression.

"What if I can't have any children?" she voiced her fears to him. "Maybe the abortion caused the miscarriage—I've read that it's possible. The neighbor was just telling me today about her friend that had four miscarriages in the last five years. . . ."

"I'm going to tell her to keep her mouth shut!" Jon shouted angrily. "What did she think she was doing—helping you?" He gritted his teeth, trying to control his temper.

Karen sighed. "They think they are, Jon. They just don't know how badly it hurts." Tears filled her eyes as she remembered another woman's comments after church the day before.

"I'm so sorry to hear about the baby, Karen," she'd said, patting Karen's hand. "But you realize, don't you, that a miscarriage is just nature's way of taking care of deformed children. . . . This is really a blessing from God." Karen had mumbled something incoherent and had hurried out the door before the lady could say anything else.

Is this a blessing from God—or a curse? Is he punishing me? she wondered. "No!" she cried, startling Jon.

"No, what?" he asked.

"I can't believe that God caused our baby to die," she said firmly. "The miscarriage happened. It just happened—and it was neither a blessing nor a curse from God." She laid her head on Jon's comforting shoulder.

"We'll have children," he said reassuringly. "Don't worry about it, Karen."

Six months later, Karen again found that she was pregnant. For a while she refused to tell anyone. She kept her hopes low, not wanting to face shattering disappointment or comments from friends again.

Fortunately, this time everything seemed normal, and at last she allowed herself to feel jubilant. She waited impatiently for that first flutter of life, but she knew long before she felt it that the baby was there, that he was part of them. She instinctively wanted to protect his life from the very beginning, and rebelled when people called the baby "it." *"It" is for things,* she reasoned. *This is a person—a him or a her. Definitely not an it!*

Karen painted the nursery a soft yellow and sewed gaily printed curtains. She frequented garage sales and secondhand stores for the items she knew their child would need. She reluctantly passed up anything that couldn't be used by either sex. "Jon, I saw the cutest little girl's dress today," she told him.

"Absolutely not! There'll be no dresses on our boy!" he teased her with a grin. "Of course, there's always the next one. . . ."

"Let's get through this experience first," she pointed out. "Then we'll see about having any more!"

The months passed too slowly for Karen. She felt awkward, heavy, and ugly, though Jon constantly assured her that she was beautiful in his eyes. The weather was unbearably hot, and their little house lacked air-conditioning.

Now, as she tossed restlessly in the middle of the night, she wondered how much longer it would be until the baby came. It was hard to be patient. Then she felt a sharp twinge, and a few minutes later, she felt the pain again. *Is it time?* she asked herself, but decided not to wake Jon until she was sure. He needed his rest, she decided.

Fifteen minutes went by and she whispered hesitantly, "Jon?"

"Wha—huh?" He sat up, looked blearily at her, and then his eyes widened in alarm. "Are you all right? Don't move!"

She giggled as she watched him frantically dash around the room. "You're so typical, Jon Hamilton," she murmured. "The absolute stereotype of the expectant father." She groaned as she felt another contraction.

Twenty minutes later, they arrived at the hospital. Throughout the long hours of her labor, Jon remained at Karen's side. "I don't think I could stand this without you," she told him.

He squeezed her hand. "I wish I could do something more to help."

Just then, everything began to happen quickly—so fast that Karen hardly realized she'd been moved to the delivery room.

"One more push!" ordered Dr. Brannigan. "Come on, Karen," he challenged her. "You can do it!"

I can't. I just can't go any further. . . . I'm too tired, Karen silently protested. Her body, drenched with sweat, felt as though a bitter war were being fought within it. The glare of the operating room lights, the uncomfortable delivery table, those abominable stirrups, and worst of all the fast, furious roller-coaster pain of labor. . . . When would it end? *Just hang on a little longer,* she told herself, choking back a scream as she felt another hard contraction.

In response, Karen gritted her teeth, and pushed with all the energy she still possessed. *The baby's coming!* she thought excitedly. A moment later, a vigorous squall shattered the air.

"No need to spank this one!" Dr. Brannigan laughed as he held up the shrieking, red-faced infant for Karen to inspect.

"Oh! She's beautiful," Karen whispered as joyful tears cascaded down her cheeks. "Can I hold her?" she asked, and reached instinctively for the baby.

"In a minute, as soon as we've checked her over," the nurse answered.

As Karen waited impatiently to hold her child, she marveled that, though weak and exhausted, her body felt so well, so whole, so light. In the last weeks of her pregnancy, Karen had often felt as though the earth's gravity had increased, making her movements heavy and plodding. Now, in delightful contrast, she experienced a euphoric sensation of weightlessness.

At last the nurse placed the now-quiet, but alert baby in Karen's arms. The infant's eyes gazed fixedly at Karen's face. *Can she see me yet? Does she know who I am?* she wondered. "Oh, you doll!" Karen scarcely breathed the words, she was so excited. "Laura, did you know that you're the most precious baby I've ever seen?"

Pride welled up within Karen. *A girl!* she thought happily. *I can't believe it!* She daydreamed about all the frilly lace and pastel-colored dresses that she'd seen hanging on department store racks. *It's definitely more fun to dress girls,* she decided as she remembered the little boys' corduroy jeans and sweatshirts that she'd also noticed on the shelves.

"Ready to head for your room?" the nurse asked Karen, breaking into her thoughts. "You have an anxious husband waiting to hear the news, too."

"Didn't you already tell him?" Karen was surprised.

"No! We figure that's your job."

"Hurry up then!" Karen begged.

The huge, double doors of the delivery room swung open as the nurses pushed Karen's bed into the hall. Karen, with tiny Laura in her arms, felt as though she were a homecoming queen riding on a parade float.

She looked up at Jon, and noted how his haggard face brightened at the sight of her and the baby. "It's a girl!" she announced.

His face beamed with pride as he kissed her. "I'll call the folks," he promised. He looked closely at his little daughter. "You're both beautiful," he said softly, and then headed for the telephone booth.

The nurses left Karen lying on the gurney in the hall while they made her bed. She turned to the infant who lay beside her. "Laura," she whispered the name almost reverently, "I can hardly believe that you're finally here—I've wanted you for such a long time."

CHAPTER

15

"WANT to go to the state fair, Karen?" Jon asked.
"I'd like to see the rodeo and go on a few rides."

"OK! That would be fun," she agreed. "I'll get
Laura ready if you'll put the stroller in the car."

They walked for miles that night, eating pop-
corn and looking at the hundreds of exhibits.
Karen was thoroughly enjoying herself when Jon
pointed across the hall.

"Isn't that one of our neighbors over there?
What's her name—Ellen?" he asked. "You should
go talk to her. She's spotted us."

Karen suddenly felt weak-kneed. "Jon, look
where she is! I can't—I just can't!" For she saw
that their neighbor was standing in front of a
prolife booth. *Maybe she'll come over here,*
Karen thought hopefully, but Ellen merely continued to smile and wave, a trifle more hesitantly
now.

"Go on, Karen. They won't bite you over

there, and Ellen's feelings are going to be hurt." He pushed the stroller and Karen firmly. "I'm with you," he said reassuringly.

But Karen's legs felt leaden as she forced herself to stand by the booth. She could barely talk and Ellen looked puzzled. As Karen tried to escape the situation, a booth worker handed her some information sheets. "I don't need information!" Karen wanted to shout at her, but of course she kept silent.

She tucked the material in a bag with the other papers she'd collected during the evening. "Can we talk someplace else?" Karen finally asked her. "This spot gives me the creeps!"

"Sure," Ellen agreed. "Abortion's a gross subject, isn't it?"

Karen hardly thought "gross" was the word to describe it, but she didn't argue. She was too thankful to move to another location. Ellen tagged along with them for several minutes, and Karen chatted comfortably.

It was late when they returned home. Karen tucked Laura into her crib, and then tossed her stack of "junk" advertisements on an empty shelf. She fell into bed exhausted.

"Did you enjoy the fair?" Jon asked as he turned off the light.

"Yes. Thanks for taking me." Neither one mentioned the prolife booth. They had already forgotten.

A few months later, Karen was busily cleaning house. She took down the lacy, white curtains to wash them, and then dusted the bookshelves. "What's up here?" she muttered as her fingers found a bunch of papers. She pulled them down to sort through the stack. "Oh goodness, from the county fair," she recalled, and sat down to skim through the free offers, advertisements, and recipes. Then her eyes fell on the prolife pamphlets.

Karen wanted to toss them into the wastebasket, but for some inexplicable reason, she set them aside. She continued to thumb through the papers, but her eyes kept returning to the prolife material. Almost against her will, she found herself reading it.

"Oh, God—no!" she cried as the facts, so long hidden from her, were suddenly revealed. One pamphlet showed the chronology of a human life. Karen's eyes closed and she felt nauseated as she realized what she had destroyed. The "mass of cells," as the family planning agency had called it, had possessed its own blood cells, a heart, arms, hands, fingers, legs, feet, toes, a foundation of an entire nervous system, forty pairs of muscles, regular blood flow, ears, eyes, nasal system, and a complete skeleton. Reflexes were present. In addition, brain wave patterns could be recorded, usually considered ample evidence of human thought capability. The stomach, liver, and kidneys also functioned. There were even lines in its palms. The material stated that the fetus looked like a miniature doll.

All of this only eight weeks after conception! Karen thought, horrified. She felt fresh agony and guilt as she realized the truth. *I killed my baby—he was real, alive—not at all what they told me he was!* she told herself, weeping.

"Oh, God, I can't stand it!" she cried. She felt as though a terrible sea monster had dredged her sin-box up from the deep ocean, and had thrown it, covered with slimy weeds, at her feet.

Jon came home that evening to find her sobbing on their bed. "Karen, what is it? What happened?" he asked. "Has something terrible happened to one of our friends?"

Karen shook her head, unable to explain the tragedy she'd just discovered.

"Is it someone in our family? Karen, tell me!"

"I didn't know, Jon. I didn't know," she repeated over and over as she wept brokenly. "Nobody ever told me!"

"Told you what? What are you talking about?" he asked, his voice edged with fright. "Karen, calm down and tell me what's going on!"

Wordless, she handed him the abortion pamphlet. His face paled as he read it and realized what they had done. He gathered her into his arms and tried to comfort her. "I didn't know, either," he said woodenly. "I didn't know."

Karen's face became drawn and haggard from lack of rest and the burden she carried. All joy was gone. She could think only of the terrible deed she'd done. *If I'd only known,* she thought, *I would never have consented to an abortion. Why did they lie to me?* The family planning agency—what a mockery of a name!—the hospital, the district attorney, Welfare. Any of them could have told her what she was really destroying! Once again, Karen's ignorance had hurt her. This time, the pain seemed excruciating.

The nightmares began. . . .

Darkness. Total darkness. She could hear the steady thump, thump, thump of a heartbeat. "Is it mine?" she wondered as she listened. And then without warning, it stopped. Period. The end.

"Start, will you?" she screamed silently from paralyzed vocal chords. "Am I dead? Am I dead, God? I can't hear you, God. Can you hear me? Is this what hell is?

"Total separation—there's no one here. I'm alone, God, and nobody cares. Nobody shares this with me. It's dark—and I'm afraid. It's silent—the heartbeat stopped—and it will never start again."

And then somehow she knew. The nurse was wrong—dead wrong. The part that hurt worst wasn't over. It never would be, nor could God answer her prayer. She would always feel, and she would always remember—it had stopped. Period. The end.

So final.

"God, is that my sentence?" she sobbed, and then as she felt the black silence closing in, suffocating her, she cried out—long, terrified screams from a shattered soul. "Oh, God," she sobbed, "I can't take it. I can't take it anymore!"

"Karen! Karen, wake up!" Jon whispered as he gently shook her awake. She opened her eyes and saw that his face reflected some of the fear that she felt inside.

"Jon, it was so terrible!" she cried. "I'm afraid! I don't want to go to sleep ever again!"

"You have to," he insisted. "You're ruining your health. You won't be able to take care of Laura if—" He stopped when he saw her agony.

"I'm sorry, honey," he apologized. "It's not your fault. I wish I knew how to get rid of those terrible dreams." He put his arms around her as if to shield her. But even as Jon slipped back into a troubled sleep, Karen lay awake.

And the nightmares grew worse. Jon prayed for her and held her tightly, but Karen continued to suffer.

"Dear God," she prayed in desperation one afternoon, "I can't live any longer without your peace. There has to be an answer. Please restore my soul, because no matter how much I want to, I can't go back and make a better choice." Karen knew she needed God's help to cope with the devastating knowledge of what she had done.

That night, she fell into a deep, restful sleep. No nightmares haunted her. Instead, God spoke to her in a beautiful dream. She saw her own concept of heaven—lots of green, grassy meadows filled with flowers, light, laughter, music . . . and then she recognized Jon playing with Laura and—she held her breath—she counted two other tiny children playing with them, too. Karen could hear their happy laughter.

Then she woke, and lay peacefully as she pondered the meaning of her dream. Before long, she understood what God was trying to say to her. It was no awful premonition that she would lose Jon and Laura in an accident—nothing like that. She believed that God was showing her a special preview: When she arrived in heaven, she'd find her other two children there, well-cared for and much-loved by her heavenly Father.

The fact that two tiny children played with Jon and Laura was important to Karen. Her nightmares had not been caused by her miscarriage; she had been able to accept and live with that loss. How like God, she thought, to provide total comfort and assurance.

"Wake up, Jon!" she exclaimed. "Something wonderful has happened, and I can't wait until morning!" She told him about her dream. "It is biblical, isn't it, Jon? The Bible says that God knows us before we are even formed in the womb. He also says that he watches over the sparrows, and knows when they fall—and he cares even more for his own children."

They agreed that it was within the nature of God to make provision for their children, both born and unborn. If their babies had complete bodies, no matter how tiny and doll-like, then surely God had given them each a soul, the most important part.

God had answered Karen's prayer. Although she would always feel sorrow and would bear scars, at last she had complete, eternal peace—his peace.

Other Living Books Bestsellers

DAVID AND BATHSHEBA by Roberta Kells Dorr. Was Bathsheba an innocent country girl or a scheming adulteress? What was King David really like? Solomon—the wisest man in the world—was to be king, but could he survive his brothers' intrigues? Here is an epic love story which comes radiantly alive through the art of a fine storyteller. 07–0618 $4.50.

TOO MEAN TO DIE by Nick Pirovolos with William Proctor. In this action-packed story, Nick the Greek tells how he grew from a scrappy immigrant boy to a fearless underworld criminal. Finally caught, he was imprisoned. But something remarkable happened and he was set free—truly set free! 07–7283 $3.95.

FOR WOMEN ONLY. This bestseller gives a balanced, entertaining, diversified treatment of all aspects of womanhood. Edited by Evelyn and J. Allan Petersen, founder of Family Concern. 07–0897 $3.95.

FOR MEN ONLY. Edited by J. Allan Petersen, this book gives solid advice on how men can cope with the tremendous pressures they face every day as fathers, husbands, workers. 07–0892 $3.50.

ROCK. What is rock music really doing to you? Bob Larson presents a well-researched and penetrating look at today's rock music and rock performers. What are lyrics really saying? Who are the top performers and what are their life-styles? 07–5686 $2.95.

THE ALCOHOL TRAP by Fred Foster. A successful film executive was about to lose everything—his family's vacation home, his house in New Jersey, his reputation in the film industry, his wife. This is an emotion-packed story of hope and encouragement, offering valuable insights into the troubled world of high pressure living and alcoholism. 07–0078 $2.95.

LET ME BE A WOMAN. Best selling author Elisabeth Elliot (author of *THROUGH GATES OF SPLENDOR*) presents her profound and unique perspective on womanhood. This is a significant book on a continuing controversial subject. 07–2162 $3.50.

WE'RE IN THE ARMY NOW by Imeldia Morris Eller. Five children become their older brother's "army" as they work together to keep their family intact during a time of crisis for their mother. 07–7862 $2.95.

WILD CHILD by Mari Hanes. A heartrending story of a young boy who was abandoned and struggled alone for survival. You will be moved as you read how one woman's love tames this boy who was more animal than human. 07–8224 $2.95.

THE SURGEON'S FAMILY by David Hernandez with Carole Gift Page. This is an incredible three-generation story of a family that has faced danger and death—and has survived. Walking dead-end streets of violence and poverty, often seemingly without hope, the family of David Hernandez has struggled to find a new kind of life. 07–6684 $2.95.

The books listed are available at your bookstore. If unavailable, send check with order to cover retail price plus 10% for postage and handling to:

Tyndale House Publishers, Inc.
Box 80
Wheaton, Illinois 60189

Prices and availability subject to change without notice. Allow 4–6 weeks for delivery.